Fluids and Electrolytes
Clinical Problems and Their Solutions

Fluids and Electrolytes

Clinical Problems and Their Solutions

Patricia A. Gabow, M.D. *Associate Professor of Medicine, University of Colorado Health Sciences Center, Denver, Colorado; Director, Department of Medicine, Denver General Hospital*

Little, Brown and Company, Boston/Toronto

Copyright © 1983 by Patricia A. Gabow

First Edition

All rights reserved. No part of this book may be reproduced in any form or by any electronic or mechanical means, including information storage and retrieval systems, without permission in writing from the publisher, except by a reviewer who may quote brief passages in a review.

Library of Congress Catalog Card No. 82-83348

ISBN 0-316-30114-0

Printed in the United States of America

SEM

To the patients who provided the clinical problems for this book, and to my husband, for his loving support in all things

Contents

Preface ix

1. Urinalysis   1

2. Acute Renal Failure   9
   Specific Patient Problem   18

3. Metabolic Acidosis   23
   Specific Patient Problems   29

4. Metabolic Alkalosis   43
   Specific Patient Problem   48

5. Hyponatremia   57
   Specific Patient Problems   62

6. Hyperosmolar States   69
   Specific Patient Problem   72

7. Disorders of Potassium Metabolism   77
   Specific Patient Problems   83

8. Disorders of Calcium Metabolism   91
   Specific Patient Problems   101

9. Disorders of Phosphorus Metabolism   107
   Specific Patient Problems   111

10. Disorders of Magnesium Metabolism   115
    Specific Patient Problems   118

Index   123

Preface

In these times of routine chemistry determinations, virtually all hospitalized patients undergo these tests. Therefore, every physician, regardless of his or her subspecialty, should be able to interpret correctly the data obtained from these routine determinations and to make appropriate therapeutic decisions from them.

This book grew out of an effort to communicate to medical students the essential concepts of fluid and electrolyte management that are used in understanding the results obtained from routine serum chemistry measurements and arterial blood gas analysis. Although originally planned for medical students, it seemed to fulfill a need to accomplish this goal for interns, residents, fellows, and practicing physicians as well.

The chapters in the book are divided into two main sections. The first section deals with factual materials on a given subject. The questions posed in this first section are best answered by reading the references suggested at the end of the chapter. The second section of each chapter centers on clinical problems. The questions posed in the second section are ones that arise in day-to-day patient management. They will serve to test how completely the factual material has been understood. Thus, if one cannot effectively manage the patient(s) presented in the second section of each chapter, more time should be spent in understanding the material presented in the first section, for the physician's knowledge is meaningful only if it can be applied to treating patients correctly and effectively.

P. A. G.

1. Urinalysis

A few months careful study in the wards of a hospital and in the deadhouse will serve to convince any unprejudiced person that the nature of renal disease may be diagnosed in many cases by the microscopial character of the urinary deposit.

Dr. Lionel S. Beale, 1852

Questions

1. What colors can a urine sample be, and what do these colors indicate pathologically?
2. How is specific gravity helpful in the clinical evaluation of a patient? What is the correlation between specific gravity and osmolality? In a hospital setting, what is the most common cause for a high specific gravity with a markedly lower osmolality?
3. What is the pH of an essentially bicarbonate-free urine; of a maximally acidified urine? What clinical information can be obtained from a dipstick test for urine pH?
4. a. What proteins are detected by the urine dipstick test for protein?
   b. A 50-year-old woman was admitted with anemia and hypercalcemia. Urinalysis by the medical student revealed no protein. The laboratory, however, using sulfosalicylic acid, reported 3+ protein in the same urine sample. How do you interpret these findings? What gives you a false positive test for albumin?
   c. A diabetic patient was referred for evaluation of proteinuria. In reviewing the old chart to determine the probable onset of proteinuria, one needs to correlate what other variable on the urinalysis with the protein?
5. What does the urine dipstick test for blood detect? How can these possible causes be differentiated?
6. What substances are detected by the urine dipstick test for ketones? In what clinical situations do urine ketones underestimate the degree of ketoacidosis? Why? In what clinical settings can positive serum ketones overestimate the amount of ketoacids?
7. What is measured by the glucose dipstick test? In what clinical settings does glucosuria occur?
8. What cellular elements can be identified in a urinalysis? How many of each type can be seen in a normal urinalysis? How does one interpret an abnormal number?
9. How should one obtain, save, and prepare a urine specimen to look for casts? What casts can be found in a urine specimen, and how should they be interpreted?
10. What urinary crystals can be seen that help in establishing a clinical diagnosis?

2 Urinalysis

Solutions to Questions

1. The following colors of a urine sample reflect the causes listed below:

Color	Abnormality or Cause
Red	Hematuria
	Hemoglobin
	Myoglobin (muscle pigment)
	Beets
	Rifampin
Orange	Bilirubin
	Pyridium (urinary analgesic used in treating cystitis)
Brown	Hemoglobin (in acid urine)
	Myoglobin
	Bilirubin
Magenta	Porphyria (on exposure to air)
Black	Alcaptonuria (on exposure to air)
	Metastatic malignant melanoma (on exposure to air, due to melanin pigment)
	Blackwater fever (hemoglobinuria from malaria)
White (milk-colored)	Chyluria; most common cause in the world is filariasis; in the U.S., pulmonary tuberculosis or a pulmonary tumor obstructing the thoracic duct

2. Since specific gravity gives a rough estimate of the concentration of the urine, this measurement should be used to assess appropriate water handling by a patient. The most accurate measurement of urinary concentration, however, is measured osmolality. The lack of correlation of specific gravity and osmolality is due to the fact that specific gravity reflects not only numbers but also density of particles, whereas osmolality is a colligative property and reflects only the number of particles.

    In a hospital setting, intravenous contrast material is probably the most frequent cause of a marked dissociation of specific gravity and osmolality. This cause should certainly be considered when specific gravity exceeds what is normally seen physiologically, that is, 1.030.

3. The pH of a bicarbonate-free urine is 6.0 or less; a maximally acidified urine is 4.5 to 5.0.

    The following clinical information can be obtained from urine pH:

    a. To evaluate appropriate acidification: It is important to recognize that the urine dipstick test for pH is not very accurate; if measurement of pH is indicated to verify appropriate renal acidification, pH by meter should be obtained of a freshly voided urine specimen. The patient who has hyperchloremic acidosis without a history of diarrhea (see Chap. 3) should always have urine pH measured to ascertain if the urine is appropriately acidified, that is, less than 5.5. Urine pH greater than 5.5 in the presence of metabolic acidosis and acidemia supports a diagnosis of distal renal tubular acidosis (see Chap. 3). This focuses attention, then, on the kidney rather than the gastrointestinal tract as the site of HCO_3 loss.

b. To follow therapy: For example, in the treatment of a sodium chloride–responsive metabolic alkalosis, HCO_3 should start to be excreted. Thus, when urine pH exceeds 6.1, euvolemia is being approached and the excess HCO_3 is being excreted.

   In certain clinical situations such as salicylate and phenobarbital intoxication, alkalization promotes excretion of these substances. As HCO_3 is administered, urine pH should be checked and should be greater than 7.0 in this setting.

   c. To assess urinary tract disease: Urine pH of 8.0 in a patient should raise the question of an infection with urea-splitting organisms such as *Proteus* organisms. A consistently acid pH in a patient with uric acid stones may promote the stone formation. Similarly, in a patient with multiple myeloma, acid urine may contribute to the development of myeloma kidney.

4. a. The urine dipstick test for protein detects albumin only. It does not detect amino acids, globulins, tubular protein (Tamm-Horsfall protein), or myeloma protein (Bence Jones protein). The last is of particular clinical importance in that a negative dipstick test in a patient with multiple myeloma does not exclude the possibility of substantial Bence Jones proteinuria.

   b. This patient probably has multiple myeloma. If the patient has Bence Jones proteinuria, the medical student would get a negative test for protein using the dipstick, and the laboratory, using sulfosalicylic acid precipitation, would get a positive test, since this method detects all proteins. A very alkaline urine will give a false positive test on albumin. The color change on the dipstick is dependent on the electrical charges on the albumin molecule, and a high pH affects this charge and results in some color change. However, this should never be the reason for 3+ and 4+ protein on urinalysis.

   c. In assessing the significance of "dipstick proteinuria," it must be emphasized that this reflects protein concentration and not the absolute amount of protein in the urine. A dipstick value for protein needs to be interpreted in relation to urine specific gravity. For example, a trace or 1+ protein determination in a urine specimen with high specific gravity may represent insignificant proteinuria, whereas 1+ in a urine sample with specific gravity of 1.005 may reflect significant proteinuria.

5. The urine dipstick test for hemoglobin detects hemoglobin and myoglobulin. Myoglobulin is a heme pigment and is measured by the orthotolidine reaction on the dipstick.

   If a patient has dipstick-positive urine with no red blood cells (RBCs) seen on microscopic examination, either the patient has hemoglobinuria or myoglobinuria. These two can generally be differentiated by looking at serum. With hemoglobinuria the serum is pigmented, and with myoglobinuria the serum is clear. This occurs because hemoglobin is only filtered after the haptoglobin has been saturated and free hemoglobin appears; myoglobulin is less protein-bound, is a significantly smaller molecule (one-fourth the size of hemoglobin), and is therefore filtered. Thus, looking at the serum for pigmentation is very helpful.

6. The urine dipsticks, "ketosticks," and Acetest tablets all measure acetoacetic acid, 3-hydroxybutyric (3-OH butyric) acid, and acetone. However, the sensitivity for acetoacetic acid is many times that for 3-OH butyric acid and acetone. Therefore, even high levels of the latter compounds may not be reflected in determinations by Acetest reactions. This is important in three clinical situations:
   a. Alcoholic ketoacidosis (AKA)
   b. Combined diabetic ketoacidosis (DKA) and lactic acidosis
   c. Recovery from ketoacidosis

   Alcoholic ketoacidosis occurs in alcoholic patients. The usual history is that of a recent "binge" followed by several days of nausea, vomiting, and no food intake. The patient presents with an anion gap metabolic acidosis and may have no or barely detectable ketones by dipstick or Acetest and high levels of 3-OH butyric acid (see Chap. 3). The state in which the ketoacids exist is determined by the redox state of the mitochondria, that is, the NADH/NAD ratio.

$$\text{Acetoacetic acid} \xrightleftharpoons{\text{NADH/NAD}} \text{3-OH butyric acid}$$

With glucose and phosphorus administration, recovery begins, the anion gap decreases, the serum bicarbonate concentration increases, and the measured serum ketones may rise. With recovery, the NADH/NAD ratio is reduced, and 3-OH butyric acid is shifted to acetoacetic acid. Therefore, one can actually see increasing ketonemia as measured by Acetest while the anion gap is decreasing and the serum bicarbonate concentration is increasing. For example:

	Initial	6 Hours
Sodium	135 mEq/L	137 mEq/L
Potassium	4.0 mEq/L	3.5 mEq/L
Bicarbonate	7 mEq/L	12 mEq/L
Chloride	100 mEq/L	102 mEq/L
Anion gap	28 mEq/L	23 mEq/L
Acetone	Trace at 1 : 1	1 : 4

Therefore, to make the diagnosis of AKA one must realize that measured ketones do not reflect 3-OH butyric acid levels. One must also be careful not to interpret the apparent increase in serum ketones as a worsening clinical condition, rather than as recovery and ketoacid conversion.

Diabetic patients are prone not only to DKA but also to lactic acidosis. In those patients where both occur, the NADH/NAD ratio is increased in both the cytoplasm (shifting pyruvate to lactate) and the mitochondria (shifting acetoacetic acid to 3-OH butyric acid). Therefore, they will have decreased Acetest measurements for the level of ketonemia; the Acetest dilution may well increase with recovery. Acetest may remain positive in DKA after the anion gap has normalized because acetone is present for 48 to 72 hours.

7. The glucose dipstick test measures only glucose, since it is impregnated with glucose oxidase. The Clinitest tablets measure all reducing sugars. Glucose is handled by the kidney by filtration and reabsorption; therefore, glucose could appear in the urine either because filtered load is increased, exceeding a normal tubular reabsorptive capacity, or because the tubular capacity to reabsorb glucose has been reduced. The increased filtered load results from hyperglycemia and from increased glomerular filtration rate; the latter occurs in pregnancy. The reduced tubular capacity to reabsorb glucose occurs with renal glucosuria of the decreased threshold or increased splay type, proximal renal tubular acidosis, and some parenchymal renal diseases.

    It is important to recognize these nonhyperglycemic causes of glucosuria, since in the absence of hyperglycemia, no insulin or oral hypoglycemic agents should be given for treatment of the glucosuria.

8. Epithelial cells of several types can be seen in a urinalysis. A few transitional epithelial cells can be seen in any normal urinalysis. These cells are two to four times the size of white blood cells (WBCs) and are usually pear-shaped or spindle-shaped. Large numbers suggest abnormal cell desquamation as may occur with inflammation or a tumor.

    Squamous epithelial cells are large, flat cells, originating from the urethra and vagina. A large number of these cells in a urine specimen obtained from a female suggests vaginal contamination of the specimen, and in that circumstance correct interpretation of RBCs, WBCs, bacteria, and culture is not possible.

    Renal tubular epithelial cells (RTCs) are large cells, one-third larger than WBCs, with clear, eccentric nuclei. Like all epithelial surfaces, the renal epithelial surface does have cell turnover, and therefore, an occasional RTC in a urinalysis is not abnormal. If one sees sheets or casts of these cells, the diagnosis of acute renal failure should be entertained.

Red blood cells can be seen in the urine. One to two RBCs per high-power field are within normal limits. More than this number are pathologic. RBCs in the urine can represent bleeding from any point in the urinary tract, from the urethral meatus to the renal parenchyma. In addition, systemic coagulation abnormalities can result in hematuria. Therefore, a patient with isolated hematuria requires investigation of the coagulation system and the entire urinary tract.

One to five WBCs per high-power field are within normal limits. Numbers in excess of this amount are pathologic. WBCs in the urine represent inflammation anywhere in the urinary tract, from the urethra to the parenchyma. It is important to note that this reflects inflammation, not infection. For example, pyuria could occur from chemical cystitis (bubble bath cystitis in young girls), acute interstitial nephritis from drugs, and acute exudative glomerulonephritis like poststreptococcal glomerulonephritis.

9. Cast: "A urinary cast is a readable message from the nephrons. Formed elements in casts are labelled as coming from the parenchyma of the kidney with a certitude that is rare in other laboratory tests" [1]. Urine to be examined for casts should be a freshly voided morning specimen. It should be spun in a conical test tube at medium speed for 3 minutes. The supernatant should be gently drained off and the button of material carefully withdrawn with a pipette and placed on a slide. Casts are best preserved in a cold, acid urine.

One can see casts of all the cellular elements listed above in #8 except for transitional and squamous epithelial cells. Casts localize the pathologic process to the kidney. An RTC cast raises questions of acute renal failure; RBC casts mean glomerulonephritis. WBC casts indicate inflammation in the kidney. A number of noncellular casts can also be seen.

Hyaline casts are difficult to see under a microscope, being essentially the same refractile index as the glass. They are composed of serum proteins. Four to five in a urinalysis can be normal. Numbers in excess of this are seen in states such as dehydration with low urine flow rates and in heavy proteinuria.

Granular casts, as the name implies, are composed of granules in a matrix, Tamm-Horsfall (tubular) protein; the granules are composed of a wide variety of serum proteins. In general, these do not connote a specific pathologic process, but rather a low urine flow rate.

Waxy casts look like slices of paraffin. They are yellowish in color and are highly refractile. Their exact origin is unclear, but they are seen in chronic renal failure.

Broad casts are formed in collecting tubules and can be any type, that is, hyaline, granular, and so forth. They occur when there is decreased function, and therefore decreased flow, in a collecting tubule draining many nephrons and hence are compatible with severe renal failure.

10. The crystals to recognize for diagnostic purposes are calcium oxalate, cystine, uric acid, and hippuric acid.

    Many calcium oxalate crystals or hippuric acid crystals in the urine of a patient with severe anion gap metabolic acidosis should suggest ethylene glycol intoxication (see Chap. 3). Many calcium oxalate crystals in other patients suggest disorders of calcium and/or oxalate metabolism.

    Cystine crystals in a patient with stones would suggest cystinuria.

    Uric acid crystals, of course, occur normally, but in patients with stone diathesis or acute renal failure, hyperuricosuria should be considered.

Reference

1. Schreiner, G. E. *Urinary Sediments.* New York: Med Com, 1969.

2. Acute Renal Failure

General Questions

1. Define *acute renal failure* (ARF).
2. In what clinical setting(s) does the question of ARF most commonly arise?
3. In this setting(s), there are three other major pathophysiologic events that must be considered in addition to ARF. What are they?
4. List the most common causes for the renal dysfunction in each of the four major categories.
5. What data from the history, symptoms, and signs may be helpful in distinguishing among prerenal azotemia (PRA), obstructive uropathy (OU), chronic renal failure (CRF), and ARF? What laboratory data may be helpful in identifying the specific ongoing disease processes involved? Construct a table.
6. What findings from urinalysis may be helpful in distinguishing among the four major categories? Construct a table.
7. What serum chemistries may be helpful in distinguishing among PRA, OU, CRF, and ARF? Comment specifically on hematocrit, serum electrolytes, calcium, and phosphorus.
8. Make a table of urinary chemistries and their characteristic values in ARF and PRA.
9. Are any radiographic examinations helpful in distinguishing among any of the four diagnostic possibilities?
10. Are there any instances in which a patient can have ARF and not be oliguric? What diagnosis should be considered in the patient who is totally anuric?
11. What is the natural history of ARF?
12. What are the complications of ARF and the mechanisms of these complications?
13. What are the aims and therapeutic modalities utilized in conservative management of ARF?
14. What are the indications for dialysis therapy in a patient with ARF?
15. What is meant by *prophylactic dialysis*?

Solutions to General Questions

1. Acute renal failure (ARF) is the rapid deterioration of renal function associated with the accumulation of nitrogenous wastes that is not due to extrarenal factors.
2. Acute oliguria is usually the clinical setting that calls attention to the possibility of ARF. An elevated or rising blood urea nitrogen (BUN) or serum creatinine also raises the question of ARF.
3. Prerenal azotemia (PRA) in which renal perfusion is markedly decreased; postrenal azotemia, or obstructive uropathy (OU); chronic renal failure (CRF); and acute presentation of chronic disease need to be considered when a patient with diminished renal function is first seen. The last situation frequently occurs in patients who do not receive regular health care.

4. The most common causes for the renal dysfunction in each major category are as follows:
   a. Prerenal azotemia
      (1) Intravascular volume depletion
      (2) Impaired cardiac function
      (3) Peripheral vasodilation
      (4) Increased renal vascular resistance
      (5) Bilateral renal artery obstruction
   b. Obstructive uropathy
      (1) Uretheral obstruction
      (2) Bladder neck obstruction
      (3) Bilateral ureteral obstruction
   c. Chronic renal failure
      (1) Glomerular disease
      (2) Interstitial disease
      (3) Vascular disease
   d. Acute renal failure
      (1) Ischemic disorders
      (2) Nephrotoxins
      (3) Glomerulonephritis
      (4) Vascular disorders
5. The interviewer's questions should be directed toward finding a cause for one of the major categories of renal dysfunction and accompanying manifestations.

Disorder	History	Symptoms	Signs	Laboratory Data
Prerenal azotemia	Losses			
	1. Vomiting	Dizziness	Orthostatic hypotension and tachycardia (if this is not found with the patient in a sitting position, it should be assessed with the patient in an upright position)	Hypokalemia, hyperbicarbonatemia, increased BUN/ creatinine ratio[a]
	2. Diarrhea	Dizziness		Hypokalemia, hypobicarbonatemia

Disorder	History	Symptoms	Signs	Laboratory Data
	3. Diabetes mellitus, poorly controlled	Dizziness, polydipsia, polyuria	Orthostatic hypotension and tachycardia	Hyperglycemia, glucosuria
	4. Diuretic therapy	Dizziness	Orthostatic hypotension and tachycardia	Hypokalemia, hyperbicarbonatemia
	Impaired cardiac function			
	1. Congestive heart failure	Shortness of breath, paroxysmal nocturnal dyspnea, orthopnea	Peripheral edema, S_3 gallop, rales	
	2. Cardiogenic shock		Hypotension, peripheral vasoconstriction	
	Redistribution of intravascular volume			
	Hypoalbuminemia			
	1. Cirrhosis	Dizziness	Edema, ascites	Evidence of hepatic dysfunction
	2. Nephrotic syndrome	Dizziness	Orthostatic hypotension, edema, proteinuria	Proteinuria
Obstructive uropathy	Stone disease	Colicky abdominal pain, fluctuating urine output[b]	Hematuria, palpable kidneys[c]	Increased BUN/ creatinine ratio[a]
	Disease with high incidence of papillary necrosis	Colicky abdominal pain	Hematuria, tissue in urine, pyuria	
	1. Diabetes mellitus			
	2. Sickle cell disease			
	3. Analgesic abuse			
	4. Pyelonephritis (acute)			

Disorder	History	Symptoms	Signs	Laboratory Data
	Prostatic hypertrophy	Frequency, urgency, nocturia; decreased caliber of stream	Prostatic enlargement or nodules	
	Extrinsic ureteral compression		Female: abnormal pelvic examination; fixed cervix	
	1. Retroperitoneal fibrosis			
	2. Carcinoma			
	3. Lymphoma			
Chronic renal failure	Underlying disease with high association with CRF	Pruritus, metallic taste, decreased cognitive ability; peripheral neuropathic symptoms, lethargy, insomnia[d]	Yellow pigmentation, excoriations, reddened conjunctiva, pericardial function rub, peripheral neuropathy[e]	
	1. Hypertension		End-organ damage; retinopathy, cardiac hypertrophy	
	2. Diabetes mellitus		Retinopathy	
	3. Collagen vascular disease	Arthralgias, arthritis; central nervous system, hematologic, or dermatologic manifestations	Evidence of antinuclear antibody, compliment, rheumatoid factor, etc., multisystem disease	
	Past history of increased BUN, creatinine, or proteinuria			

Disorder	History	Symptoms	Signs	Laboratory Data
Acute renal failure	Prolonged prerenal state (see Prerenal azotemia) Nephrotoxins 1. Aminoglycosides 2. Contrast media			

[a] The BUN/creatinine ratio is usually 10 : 1. An increased ratio frequently occurs in prerenal azotemia and obstructive nephropathy. In these settings urine flow rates are decreased, providing a long contact time of tubular fluid with tubular epithelium. Urea diffuses back from the lumen to the peritubular capillary, decreasing urea clearance. Urea clearance decreases to a greater extent than creatinine clearance, which is not flow-dependent, due to the absence of creatinine diffusion across the tubular epithelium. However, BUN reflects not only clearance of urea but also protein intake and protein anabolic and catabolic rates. Therefore, a chronic alcoholic patient with a very low protein intake, reflecting the low protein content of Thunderbird, may have a BUN/creatinine ratio of 10 : 1 despite volume depletion. In contrast, a septic catabolic trauma victim may have a markedly increased BUN/creatinine ratio despite ARF rather than PRA.

[b] Fluctuations from polyuria to anuria are almost pathognomonic for OU.

[c] In addition, palpable kidneys can occur in any instance in which renal edema occurs, e.g., acute obstruction, acute glomerulonephritis, and acute renal vein thrombosis.

[d] Symptoms of CRF.

[e] Physical findings of CRF.

6. The following table illustrates certain findings from urinalysis that are helpful in distinguishing among the major categories of renal dysfunction.

Element	Prerenal Azotemia	Obstructive Uropathy	Chronic Renal Failure	Acute Renal Failure
Dipstick proteinuria ≥3+	No	No	Yes, in glomerulonephritis (GN)	Yes, in rapidly progressive GN (RPGN)
Heme +; no red blood cells (RBCs)	No	No	No	Yes, in rhabdomyolysis or hemolysis-related ARF
RBCs >10–15/ high-power field (HPF)	No	Yes, in intrinsic obstruction, e.g., stone	Yes, in chronic GN	Yes, in renal artery embolism, renal vein thrombosis; RPGN
White blood cells (WBCs) >10–15/ HPF	No	Yes, in papillary necrosis or obstruction with infection	Yes, in chronic interstitial nephritis	Yes, in RPGN; acute interstitial nephritis
Renal tubular cells >10–15/ HPF	No	No	No	Yes
Hyaline cast (many)	No	No	Yes	Only in some RPGN
Granular cast (many)	Yes	Yes	Yes	Yes; may be pigmented
Muddy-brown granular cast	No	No	No	Yes, renal failure casts
RBC casts	No	No	Yes, in GN	In RPGN only
WBC casts	No	If associated with pyelonephritis	Yes, in chronic interstitial nephritis	Yes, in acute interstitial nephritis

Note: A totally benign urinalysis suggests extrinsic urinary tract obstruction.

7. There are no serum chemistries that have any high degree of specificity in distinguishing acute from chronic renal failure, or these two disorders from pre- or postrenal azotemia. However, alterations in serum values may be more suggestive for one entity than for the other.

Serum Chemistry	Prerenal Azotemia	Obstructive Uropathy	Chronic Renal Failure	Acute Renal Failure	Comments
Sodium (Na)	Not helpful	Not helpful	Not helpful	Not helpful	Hyponatremia can occur in any of these states. Markedly increased Na is most common in PRA.
Potassium (K)	Maybe ↑	↑	Maybe ↑	↑	
Bicarbonate (HCO_3)	Usually not <15 mEq/L	Maybe <10 mEq/L	12–15 mEq/L	Maybe <10 mEq/L	May be increased in PRA from metabolic alkalosis.
Anion gap	Frequently only mildly ↑	↑	20–22 mEq/L	Maybe markedly ↑↑	
BUN/creatinine	>10 : 1; BUN usually <75–100 mg/100 ml; creatinine usually <4–5 mg/100 ml	>10 : 1	10 : 1	10 : 1	See #5 under Solutions to General Problems.
Calcium (Ca)	Usually normal to high if intravascular volume depletion results in ↑ albumin	Maybe ↓	↓	May be very low in setting of ↑ phosphate (PO_4) or rhabdomyolysis	Statistically hypocalcemia is most common in CRF, but it may occur in ARF, particularly in rhabdomyolysis.
PO_4	Usually normal	↑	↑	↑ (especially rhabdomyolysis)	
Hematocrit (HCT)	Normal to high if volume depletion	Normal to low	↓	Normal to low	In ARF, HCT can decrease to 25–30% in 3 weeks.

8. The urinary chemistry values in ARF and PRA are as follows:

	ARF	PRA
Urine sodium (U_{Na})	>40 mEq/L	<20 mEq/L
Urine osmolality	<400 mOsm/kg	>500 mOsm/kg
Urine-plasma creatinine (U_{Cr}/P_{Cr})	<20	>40
Renal failure index $\left(\dfrac{U_{Na}}{U_{Cr}/P_{Cr}}\right)$	>2	<1

9. Flat plate of the abdomen is particularly helpful in distinguishing CRF from the other three diagnostic possibilities. In general, in end-stage CRF the renal size is small as opposed to PRA in which the renal outline is normal in size and ARF and OU in which the edematous kidneys may appear large. There are a number of important exceptions to this generalization, in which kidney size is normal to large in the presence of end-stage renal disease. These include polycystic kidney disease, diabetic nephropathy, tuberous sclerosis, amyloidosis, obstructive uropathy (large hydronephrotic sacs), myeloma kidney, and occasionally sarcoid nephropathy and urate nephropathy.

    Radiographic procedures are pivotal in diagnosing urinary tract obstruction. Excretory urography with nephrotomography and delayed films, retrograde urography, antigrade pyelography with a percutaneous nephrostomy, ultrasonography, and computerized axial tomography can all be utilized to evaluate the calyceal system for an obstructive pattern. The choice of procedure depends on the expertise at a given hospital, the condition of the patient, and the need to perform a diagnostic and therapeutic procedure simultaneously.

    If a diagnosis of ARF due to a vascular catastrophe is being seriously considered, a renal scan or renal arteriography should be utilized. Renal venogram is probably the best procedure if renal vein thrombosis is being considered.

10. Oliguria is not part of the definition of ARF. About 20 percent of patients with ARF have nonoliguric renal failure (24-hr urine output >1 L). This is particularly common in aminoglycoside nephrotoxicity. In the presence of total anuria, one should consider complete obstruction of the urinary tract, cortical necrosis, bilateral renal artery embolism, and occasionally, rapidly progressive glomerulonephritis.

11. In oliguric ARF the total duration of the ARF is about 3 weeks with about 2 weeks of oliguria and 1 week of recovery. The overall mortality in ARF is about 50 percent. It is higher in trauma patients and lower in obstetric patients.

12. The complications of ARF are biochemical and systemic. Biochemical complications and the mechanism for each are

Hyperkalemia	↓ excretion + ↑ catabolism
Hyperphosphatemia	↓ excretion + ↑ catabolism
Hyperuricemia	↓ excretion + ↑ catabolism
Acidosis	↓ hydrogen ion and organic acid excretion and ↑ catabolism
Hypocalcemia	↑ serum PO_4; ↓ synthesis by the kidney of 1,25-dihydroxycholecalciferol
Hyponatremia	↓ free water clearance due to ↓ glomerular filtration rate (GFR)
Hypermagnesemia	↓ excretion coupled with ↑ magnesium intake such as in antacids

Systemic complications and the mechanism for each are

Hypertension	Generally reflects ↑ salt and water
Anemia	↓ synthesis and some degree of hemolysis
Infection	↓ white cell function and ↓ immune competence in uremia
Gastrointestinal bleeding	Cause not known

Infection and gastrointestinal bleeding are the major causes of death in ARF.

13. The major aims of conservative management of ARF are to decrease the obligatory secretory load of the compromised kidney, to carefully monitor intake of "therapeutic agents" normally excreted by the kidney, and to take a preventive stance regarding the major causes of mortality and morbidity—infection and gastrointestinal bleeding.
    a. Decrease excretory load of nitrogenous waste:
       (1) Adequate caloric intake: 100 gm of glucose per day minimum is needed to prevent endogenous catabolism.
       (2) Protein restriction: 40-gm protein diet of high biologic value protein will enable positive nitrogen balance and utilization of urea nitrogen in protein synthesis.
       (3) Sodium restriction: 1- to 2-gm sodium restriction in oliguric ARF; sodium restriction may not be needed in nonoliguric ARF.
       (4) Water restriction: Water intake should be equal to output and insensible loss. Insensible loss needs to be adjusted for fever and metabolic water production. Insensible loss usually equals 500 to 700 ml per day.
       (5) Potassium restriction: No potassium should be given, and dietary intake of potassium should be low.

b. Alter drug therapy:
   (1) Stop all unnecessary drugs.
   (2) Check all drug dosages.
   Drugs contraindicated in ARF include tetracycline, as it increases the BUN; triamterene and spironolactone because of their effect to increase potassium; and nitrofurantoins, nalidixic acid, and methenamine because they are not therapeutic at reduced GFR.
c. Preventive medicine:
   (1) Remove all unnecessary intravenous lines.
   (2) Remove Foley catheter unless significant outlet obstruction is present that cannot be managed by intermittent straight catheterization.
   (3) The role of cimetidine in preventing gastrointestinal bleeding in this setting is not established. If cimetidine is used, its dose must be decreased; if antacids are used, they must not contain magnesium.
14. The indications for acute or emergency dialysis therapy in a patient with ARF are
    a. Uncontrolled fluid and electrolyte abnormalities. For example, a patient with congestive heart failure and severe acidosis could not tolerate the sodium load of bicarbonate therapy and would require dialysis.
    b. Central nervous system dysfunction, such as marked lethargy, coma, seizures, or marked asterixis.
    c. The presence of a toxic load of dialyzable drug ordinarily excreted by the kidneys; for example, salicylate intoxication in the presence of ARF.
    d. Probable indications are pericarditis and bleeding abnormalities; in the latter instance, dialysis would be utilized in an attempt to restore platelet function.
15. Prophylactic dialysis is the use of dialysis therapy prior to the presence of a complication that would require emergency dialysis. This generally is accepted to mean dialysis therapy at an interval sufficient to maintain the BUN below 100 mg/100 ml and serum creatinine below 10 mg/100 ml. Some nephrologists suggest that prophylactic dialysis should be at an interval sufficient essentially to normalize serum chemistries (predialysis BUN <50 mg/100 ml; creatinine <5 mg/100 ml). The data suggest that this may decrease the mortality and morbidity of ARF secondary to trauma.

Specific Patient Problem

R.B. is a 68-year-old man who was brought from a boarding home to the emergency room by ambulance. The patient had the diagnosis of schizophrenia and was a chronic alcoholic. He was thought not to have been drinking recently. Workers at the boarding home became concerned when he stopped coming to meals 6 days prior to admission. On the day of admission he was found lying on the floor of his room refusing to communicate.

Physical examination on admission revealed an elderly man in no acute distress. He refused to speak. Blood pressure was 110/50 mm Hg, pulse 100 per minute, supine; blood pressure 80/40 mm Hg, pulse 120 per minute, sitting; temperature 38°C; respiration 18 per minute. Skin turgor was decreased. Neck veins were not apparent with the patient supine. Both elbows and knees showed evidence of pressure necrosis. The remainder of the physical was normal except for mental status, which could not be tested.

The patient's initial laboratory values were as follows:

HCT	42%
Na	140 mEq/L
K	4 mEq/L
Chloride (Cl)	105 mEq/L
HCO_3	16 mEq/L
BUN	41 mEq/L
Glucose	155 mEq/L

1. What are the four possible considerations for the patient's elevated BUN? What data from the history and physical examination support each diagnosis?
2. During the first 2 hours the patient was in the hospital he had no urine output. What would you do diagnostically and therapeutically at this time? Write the initial intravenous therapy orders.
3. What further laboratory data, if any, would you order at this time?
4. The patient was given 3 liters of normal saline, resulting in an increase in supine blood pressure to 120/80 mm Hg, a decrease in supine pulse to 85 beats per minute, and a decrease in orthostatic hypotension. Trace pitting edema also occurred in the lower extremities, particularly the thighs. Insertion of the Foley catheter yielded 50 ml of urine. Urinalysis revealed 3+ hemoglobin, 2+ protein, 1+ ketones, 0 glucose, no RBCs, no WBCs, and numerous pigmented casts. The patient excreted no urine with the Foley catheter in place during the 2 hours in which normal saline was given, and intravascular volume was restored. Additional laboratory data were not yet available. What would you do therapeutically at this point?
5. Laboratory data then became available and revealed:

Calcium	8.3 mg/100 ml
Phosphorus	3.4 mg/100 ml
Albumin	4.0 mg/100 ml
Uric acid	10.6 mg/100 ml
Creatinine	3.0 mg/100 ml
Lactic dehydrogenase (LDH)	2,175 IU
Serum glutamic oxaloacetic transaminase (SGOT)	900 IU
Creatinine phosphokinase (CPK)	44,000 IU
U_{Na}	86 mEq/L
Urine osmolality	280 mOsm

What are your diagnoses at this point? What data support them?

6. How would you manage the patient at this point? What would be your orders for diet, fluids, Foley catheter care, intravenous therapy, and repeat laboratory data? What other clinical data would you follow?
7. On the second hospital day, the patient was still severely oliguric (24-hr urine output <200 ml). The following laboratory data were obtained:

HCT	23%
Na	140.0 mEq/L
K	4.8 mEq/L
HCO_3	20.0 mEq/L
Cl	100.0 mEq/L
BUN	70.0 mEq/L
Creatinine	9.2 mEq/L
Uric acid	12.0 mEq/L

   What would your management include at this point?
8. On the twenty-third hospital day, the nurses' notes recorded that the patient had been incontinent of urine four times. What does this suggest to you? What action would you take?

Solutions to Specific Patient Problem

1. a. Prerenal azotemia
   b. Obstructive uropathy
   c. Chronic renal failure
   d. Acute renal failure

   The patient's history of no food intake, orthostatic hypotension, flat neck veins in the supine position, and poor skin turgor are compatible with intravascular volume depletion, which could produce PRA. Since the patient is known to be schizophrenic, it is possible he is on medication such as phenothiazines, which can produce orthostatic hypotension. However, these medications do not decrease the intravascular volume (decreased neck vein fullness) or decrease the skin turgor. Obstructive uropathy from prostatic hypertrophy should be considered when a patient is first seen and no previous data exist. Acute renal failure must be considered. The most common cause of ARF is prolonged PRA, which this patient apparently had. In addition, he may well have had rhabdomyolysis, since he was found on the floor with areas of pressure necrosis. Rhabdomyolysis is a major cause of ARF, particularly in the setting of intravascular volume depletion.

2. Although PRA may not have been the sole cause of the patient's elevated BUN, his intravascular volume was certainly depleted. Therefore, the initial intervention should be directed at reestablishing intravascular volume. In a patient who has not suffered blood loss or who is not severely anemic, this is best accomplished with normal saline. In this patient, one can give 500 ml of normal saline over the first half hour and then reevaluate. The appearance of neck veins and/or the appearance of rales should be the end point. Ordinarily in such a patient, loss of orthostatic hypotension is the best sign to use as an end point. This may be less helpful in a patient on phenothiazine therapy; however, it should still be followed. No potassium should be added to the intravenous fluids until a urine output is established or hypokalemia occurs. A Foley catheter should be passed to evaluate the patient for bladder outlet obstruction. The absence of a percussible bladder on physical examination is not sufficiently sensitive to exclude this possibility. Any urine obtained should be used for urinalysis as well as for determination of sodium, creatinine, and osmolality.
3. A serum creatinine should be obtained, since this is a better reflection of the GFR than is BUN, which is affected by protein load, catabolic states, and urine flow rate. Given the fact that the patient was found on the floor and had areas of pressure necrosis, serum should be analyzed for serum glutamic oxaloacetic transaminase (SGOT), lactic dehydrogenase (LDH), creatine phosphokinase (CPK), calcium, phosphorus, and uric acid. The CPK, SGOT, LDH, and phosphorus rise in rhabdomyolysis, reflecting the release of these substances from damaged muscle. Calcium may be low and uric acid very high.
4. The use of furosemide or mannitol to obtain a urine output should be considered. There are no controlled prospective data that demonstrate that the use of these agents early in the course of ARF alters the course of the illness. However, there are experimental data that show that establishment of a vigorous diuresis prior to a renal insult will prevent or attenuate ARF. In addition, some clinical studies suggest that the use of these agents may convert oliguric ARF to nonoliguric ARF, a disorder with a more benign course. Given the suggestive data and the relative safety of a furosemide therapy, it would seem advisable to attempt to establish a urine output using this agent. Initially, 1 mg of furosemide per kilogram can be given, followed in 1 hour by 2 mg per kilogram, and then 5 mg per kilogram if no response occurs. It does not seem to be efficacious to exceed that dose. Mannitol could be utilized in place of furosemide, but its effect to increase intravascular volume acutely may not be desirable in some patients who have already achieved euvolemia by fluid therapy.

5. The patient had (a) rhabdomyolysis. He was found on the floor with areas of pressure necrosis; he had orthotolidine-positive urine without RBCs and clear serum; he had increased CPK, LDH, and SGOT. The absence of hyperkalemia and hyperphosphatemia suggests that he may have been hypokalemic and hypophosphatemic prior to the rhabdomyolysis, both of which are common in malnourished, alcoholic individuals. In fact, they may have contributed to the muscle necrosis. (b) Oliguric ARF. The urine sodium was greater than 40 mEq per liter, urine osmolality was less than 400 mOsm, urine-plasma creatinine ratio was less than 20, and renal failure index (RFI) was greater than 2.
6. Substances ordinarily excreted by the kidney must be limited in patients with oliguric renal failure. The patient should be placed on a 40-gm protein (high biologic value protein), 2-gm sodium, low-potassium diet. Fluid intake should be restricted to losses plus insensible loss. The latter equals about 500 to 700 ml per day. Intravenous therapy is not necessary, and all unnecessary lines should be removed. Once the patient is in established ARF, it is not necessary to monitor the urine output; a variation from 200 to 400 ml per day is of little consequence. Therefore, the Foley catheter should be removed. It is probably advisable to follow daily electrolytes, creatinine, and BUN initially. Temperature; blood pressures and pulse, lying and standing (or sitting); weight, mental status, and stool Hematest should be performed in order to monitor infectious complications, intravascular volume, symptoms of uremia, and occult gastrointestinal bleeding.
7. The patient was demonstrating the rapidly rising creatinine. The patient should receive prophylactic hemodialysis. Although his BUN was below 100 mg/100 ml, the serum creatinine was over 9 mg/100 ml, and these variables were rapidly rising. The uric acid would also be lowered by dialysis. Once the patient is being hemodialyzed on a regular schedule, it might be possible or necessary to increase fluid, salt, and protein intake.
8. In a previously severely oliguric patient, this sign suggests the onset of the diuretic, or recovery phase, of ARF. It is essential that the patient be maintained euvolemic during this phase in order to facilitate recovery. Salt and fluid intake usually need to be liberalized at this juncture. Weight; blood pressures, lying and standing; and urine output need to be carefully monitored.

Suggested Reading

Anderson, R. J., et al. Non-oliguric renal failure. *N. Engl. J. Med.* 296:1134, 1977.

Miller, T. R., et al. Urinary diagnostic indices in acute renal failure: A prospective study. *Ann. Intern. Med.* 89:47, 1978.

Schrier, R. W., and Conger, J. D. Acute Renal Failure: Pathogenesis, Diagnosis, and Management. In R. W. Schrier (Ed.), *Renal and Electrolyte Disorders* (2nd ed.). Boston: Little, Brown, 1980. Pp. 375–408.

Swan, R. C., and Merrill, J. P. The clinical cause of acute renal failure. *Medicine* 23:215, 1953.

3. Metabolic Acidosis

General Questions

1. Define *metabolic acidosis*.
2. List the two broad categories of metabolic acidosis, and explain in what ways they are different pathophysiologically.
3. List the causes (endogenous and exogenous) of anion gap metabolic acidosis, name the anion responsible for the gap in each, and explain how you would diagnose each disorder. Are there causes of an increased anion gap that are not associated with metabolic acidosis?
4. List the causes of hyperchloremic acidosis, and explain how they occur.

   In order to understand renal tubular acidosis (RTA), one must first understand how the kidney originally handles bicarbonate anion (HCO_3^-) and hydrogen ion (H^+).
5. How is HCO_3^- reabsorbed in the proximal tubule? Fill in the diagram below, illustrating the reabsorption of the filtered HCO_3^-.

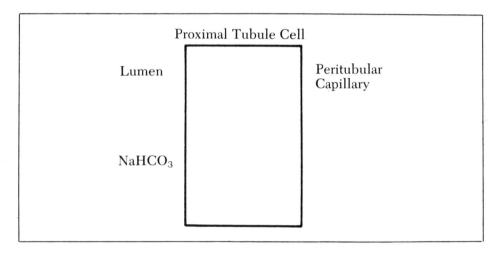

   What percentage of filtered HCO_3^- is reabsorbed in the proximal tubule? How is distal HCO_3^- reabsorption different from proximal? If all the filtered HCO_3^- were reabsorbed, would the serum HCO_3^- go up, go down, or stay the same? Why?
6. What are the differences between proximal and distal RTA in terms of renal acidification and associated abnormalities?

Solutions to General Questions

1. Metabolic acidosis is a primary pathologic process resulting in the addition of hydrogen ion or the loss of bicarbonate, which if unopposed would result in acidemia.

   It is important not to define metabolic acidosis in terms of a low serum bicarbonate concentration or systemic arterial pH because in mixed acid-base disturbances these variables may be normal or even elevated.

2. The broad categories of metabolic acidosis are anion gap metabolic acidosis and normal gap or hyperchloremic acidosis. In general terms, anion gap metabolic acidosis results from the addition of endogenous or exogenous acid, and hyperchloremic acidosis (with a few exceptions) results from the loss of bicarbonate.

   In the anion gap type of metabolic acidosis, the calculated anion gap increases. The anion gap is calculated as sodium (Na) − chloride (Cl) − bicarbonate (HCO_3). The anion gap increases because the HCO_3 is used to buffer the organic acid and the organic anion remains in the blood. For example, in ketoacidosis:

   $$\underbrace{Ketoanion + H^+}_{ketoacid} + NaHCO_3 \rightarrow H_2O + CO_2 + Na\ ketoanion$$

   Therefore, as bicarbonate is consumed, the sodium is electrically balanced by the ketoanion. Since the ketoanion is not included in the calculation for the anion gap, the calculated anion gap increases.

   In hyperchloremic acidosis, an organic acid is not added to the body; rather, HCO_3 is lost. In this instance electrical neutrality is maintained by the addition of chloride anion. Since chloride is included in the anion gap calculation, the anion gap does not increase.

3. The causes of anion gap metabolic acidosis are outlined in the following table.

Disorder	Anion	Method of Diagnosis
Endogenous		
Ketoacidosis		
Diabetic ketoacidosis	Acetoacetate (AcAc) 3-hydroxybutyrate (3HB)	Glucose >250 mg/100 ml; pH <7.2; serum ketones.
Alcoholic ketoacidosis	3HB alone in some patients; 3HB and AcAc in others	Compatible history; chronic alcoholism with recent binge associated with no food and vomiting. pH 6.9–7.7; HCO_3 low to high. Ketones present or absent. Largely diagnosed by history. (See Chap. 1.)
Starvation ketosis	AcAc 3HB	HCO_3 not <18 mEq/L and history of no food intake; serum ketones.
Lactic acidosis	Lactate	Diagnosis largely of exclusion; a clinical setting of decreased tissue oxygenation. This can be gross, as in shock, or a subtle matter at the cellular level, as in CO poisoning. 50% of clinical diagnoses of lactic acidosis are not confirmed biochemically.

Disorder	Anion	Method of Diagnosis
Renal failure	Sulfate, phosphates, and a diversity of organic acids	Elevated blood urea nitrogen (BUN) and creatinine; creatinine usually >7 mg/100 ml. In acute renal failure, acidosis occurs earlier and may be more severe depending upon catabolic rate of patient.
Hyperglycemic Hyperosmolar nonketotic coma	Unknown	Hyperosmolarity due to ↑ glucose. Mild acidosis without significant ketones.
Respiratory alkalosis	Lactate Citrate	Anion gap increased about 3–4 mEq/L.
Metabolic alkalosis	Unknown; may represent change in protein charge	Alkalemia and alkalosis plus anion gap without evidence for specific organic acid.
Exogenous		
Salicylate intoxication	Salicylate Lactate Ketones ? Others	Mixed acid-base disturbance; usually metabolic acidosis and respiratory alkalosis with alkalemia; blood salicylate level.
Methanol intoxication	Formate	Usually alcoholic patient; appears intoxicated; visual complaints; abdominal pain. Optic nerve edema, blindness (<10%); methanol level.
Ethylene glycol intoxication	Glycolate Oxalate	Frequently alcoholic patient; appears intoxicated; severe acidosis; calcium oxalate crystals or hippuric acid crystals in urine (see Chap. 1). This is an urgent diagnosis to make; blood measurements are not readily available and results are not available in patient's lifetime. The presence of an osmolar gap has been used (see Note below).
Paraldehyde overdose	?	Smell patient's breath. Test for ketones is false positive in this situation.
Phenformin	Lactate	History of phenformin treatment in acidotic diabetic without hyperglycemia or ketonemia. (Phenformin no longer commercially available in United States.)
INH overdose	Lactate	History.
Chloral hydrate overdose	Lactate	History; drug screen.
Iron overdose	?	History.

Note: Osmolar gap = measured osmolality − calculated osmolality. Calculated osmolality = 1.8 Na + 0.3 BUN + 0.06 glucose + 0.2 blood alcohol (mg/100 ml). If the difference is >15 mOsm in an acidotic patient with no other clear cause for acidosis, consider the patient to have ingested ethylene glycol and treat accordingly. Since the lethal dose is small, fatal ethylene glycol intoxication can occur without an osmolar gap.

An elevated anion gap can occur in the absence of acidosis in the following circumstances: (a) therapy with sodium salts of an organic acid, such as sodium lactate in Ringer's lactate or sodium acetate in Plasmanate or dialysate, and (b) accumulation of exogenous anion, such as salicylate, penicillin, or carbenicillin. In these settings, metabolic alkalosis can occur. In Group a, metabolic alkalosis can be produced by metabolism of the anion to form bicarbonate. In Group b, metabolic alkalosis can result by excretion of the unreabsorbable anion with potassium and ammonium with concomitant renal generation of the alkalosis.

4. The causes of hyperchloremic acidosis are outlined in the following table.

Disorder	Mechanism
Endogenous	
Diarrhea	Most common cause; loss of HCO_3 and potential HCO_3, such as citrate, in diarrheal fluid.
Renal tubular acidosis	Renal wasting of HCO_3.
Small bowel or pancreatic drainage	Loss of HCO_3 or HCO_3 equivalent from gastrointestinal tract.
Ureterosigmoidostomy; obstructed or long ileostomy	Normal intestinal absorption of sodium chloride (NaCl) and secretion of potassium bicarbonate ($KHCO_3$); occurs when mucosa is presented with a large NaCl load from the urine.
Aldosterone deficiency	$\downarrow$ ammonia production is secondary to $\uparrow K$ as well as the loss of aldosterone's direct effect on H^+ secretion.
Hyperparathyroidism	Renal HCO_3 wasting due to proximal tubular effect of parathyroid hormone.
Recovery from ketoacidosis	Excretion of the anion, leaving a low serum HCO_3 without an anion; corrects as the kidney generates "new" HCO_3 by ammonia excretion.
Exogenous	
Carbonic anhydrase inhibitor	Results in a picture indistinguishable from renal tubular acidosis. (Who takes Diamox?)[a]
Overtreatment with HCl acid; lysine HCl or arginine HCl	HCl acid—direct effect; lysine HCl and arginine HCl→HCl after deamination.
Anion exchange resins (cholestyramine)	Binds HCO_3 in gastrointestinal tract in exchange for Cl.
Certain hyperalimentation fluids	Solution that contains organic cations in excess of organic anions results in hyperchloremic acidosis since metabolism cationic amino acid yields a H^+.
Ammonium chloride (NH_4Cl)	HCl results from metabolism. (How do you find out if a patient is taking NH_4Cl? What might a patient be taking that would contain NH_4Cl?)[b]
Spironolactone	Interference with aldosterone activity directly or indirectly due to $\uparrow K^+$.

[a]Elderly patients with glaucoma are treated with Diamox. Therefore when an elderly patient enters the hospital with hyperchloremic acidosis, ask the patient if he is being treated for an eye condition.
[b]NH_4Cl is in some over-the-counter diet pills.

5. The figure below illustrates how filtered bicarbonate is resorbed in the proximal tubule.

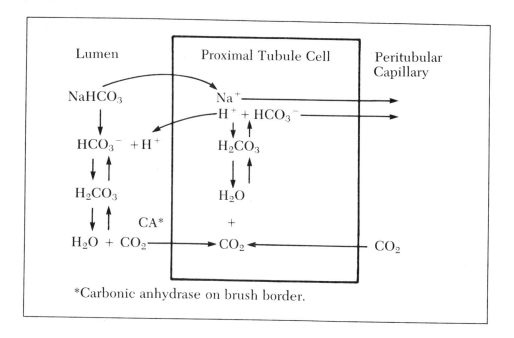

*Carbonic anhydrase on brush border.

Eighty-five to 90 percent of filtered bicarbonate is reabsorbed in the proximal tubule. Ten to 15 percent is absorbed in the distal tubule.

Because carbonic anhydrase is present in the brush border of the proximal tubule cell, carbonic acid (H_2CO_3) is promptly broken down to $H_2O + CO_2$, thereby preventing the establishment of a hydrogen ion gradient; that is, hydrogen ions are not present in any substantial amount in the lumen. Therefore, bicarbonate secretion is not limited by the membrane's ability to maintain a gradient. This makes the proximal tubule a high-capacity system; it can reabsorb a large quantity of bicarbonate but can maintain only a low gradient.

The distal tubule contains carbonic anhydrase only within the cell. Therefore, H_2CO_3 is not quickly broken down to $CO_2 + H_2O$, and a gradient for hydrogen ion is established, making the distal tubule a low-capacity, high-gradient system.

If only all the filtered bicarbonate were reabsorbed, the serum bicarbonate could not go up, since only what was filtered would be reclaimed. The serum bicarbonate would not stay constant if only that which was filtered were reabsorbed because each day in metabolism 1 mEq of acid per kilogram is generated. This acid is buffered by available bicarbonate. If this bicarbonate were not replaced, the serum bicarbonate would eventually fall.

28 Metabolic Acidosis

The kidney generates new bicarbonate by secreting hydrogen ion, which combines with sulfate (SO_4) or phosphate (PO_4) to form titratable acidity or with ammonia (NH_3) to form ammonium (NH_4).

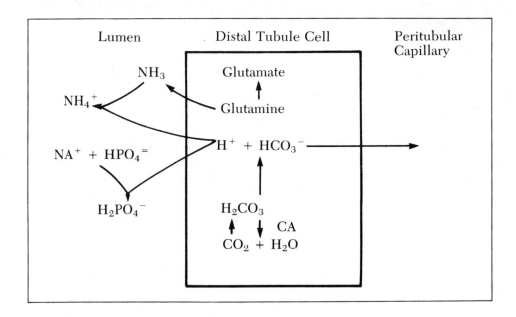

Since these hydrogen ions are not used in reclaiming a luminal bicarbonate, the bicarbonate left behind in the cell is "new" bicarbonate. This explains why acidosis occurs in clinical entities in which ammonia excretion is impaired, such as hyporeninemic hypoaldosteronism (see Specific Patient Problems, Patient A).

6. A major difference between proximal and distal renal tubular acidosis (RTA) that aids in their differentiation is that with significant acidosis and a decrease in the serum bicarbonate concentration (<12 mEq/L), patients with proximal RTA acidify their urine. Patients with distal RTA never maximally acidify their urine, even in the face of severe acidosis (urine pH > 5.5).

In proximal RTA, the reabsorptive capacity for bicarbonate in the proximal tubule is impaired. For example, in a given patient, perhaps 75 percent rather than 85 percent of the filtered bicarbonate is reabsorbed. The distal tubule then is delivered 25 percent, not 15 percent, of the filtered bicarbonate. Since the distal tubule is a low-capacity system, it is unable to reclaim the excess bicarbonate, and the anion is excreted in the urine. As the serum bicarbonate falls, the absolute amount of bicarbonate delivered distally decreases, the distal tubule has the capacity to absorb it, and the urine becomes appropriately acidic (<5.4). In distal RTA, the portion of the tubule that ordinarily reabsorbs the final molecules of bicarbonate and acidifies the urine is not maximally functional. Therefore, even in severe acidemia some bicarbonate remains, and the urine pH is not maximally acid.

Proximal RTA can be associated with inability to reabsorb substances other than bicarbonate; for example, glucose, phosphate, uric acid, and amino acids. Therefore, patients with proximal RTA can have hypophosphatemia, hypouricemia, glycosuria, and amino aciduria. Distal RTA is frequently associated with nephrocalcinosis and nephrolithiasis. These occur only in distal RTA, despite the fact that hypercalciuria occurs in both types.

RTA	Serum Bicarbonate	Urine Acidification with Acidosis	Serum Potassium
Type I (distal)	↓	Impaired	Normal (nl) or ↓
Type II (proximal)	↓	Intact	nl or ↓
Type IV (hypoaldosteronism)	↓	Intact	nl or ↑

Type IV RTA occurs in patients with modest impairment of renal function and is associated with hyperkalemia rather than hypokalemia (see Specific Patient Problems, Patient A).

Specific Patient Problems
Patient A

An elderly woman was brought to the emergency room by neighbors. She was obtunded and appeared dehydrated. She had stool and urine on her clothing. Physical examination revealed blood pressure 100/60 mm Hg, pulse 90 per minute, supine; blood pressure 70/30 mm Hg, pulse 105 per minute, with elevation of head of the bed: flat neck veins, and decreased skin turgor. Kussmaul's respiration was apparent. Neurologic examination revealed no focal signs. The patient weighed 50 kg. Laboratory studies revealed the following:

pH	7.25	K	2.5 mEq/L
PCO_2	14 mm Hg	Cl	118 mEq/L
HCO_3	5 mEq/L	Creatinine	3.4 mg/100 ml
Na	133 mEq/L	BUN	52 mg/100 ml

1. What is the acid-base disturbance? Is the compensation appropriate? What are the most likely causes?
2. What aspects of the presentation support your diagnosis?
3. How would you proceed with simple maneuvers and tests to make the diagnosis?
4. What would you anticipate the amount of potassium deficit to be: mild or moderate? Why?
5. What are possible reasons for the increased BUN and creatinine? Which of the possibilities is critical to diagnose now? How does one differentiate among these possibilities?
6. Why is the BUN disproportionately increased as compared to creatinine, that is, BUN/creatinine > 10 : 1? Explain this in terms of how urea and creatinine are handled by the kidney.
7. In general terms, what does the patient need therapeutically? What would your initial intravenous therapy orders be?

Metabolic Acidosis

8. Would you give sodium bicarbonate (NaHCO$_3$)? Why? How much would you give? Why? How would you give it? Why?
9. Would you give potassium? Why? How much and at what rate would you give it?

Patient B

J. R. is a 24-year-old diabetic requiring insulin. His diabetes was secondary to pancreatic resection for hemorrhagic pancreatitis. Three days prior to admission he developed diarrhea, vomiting, and increasing lethargy. He was brought into the emergency room semicomatose. Physical examination revealed a thin male with Kussmaul's respiration, temperature 37°C, blood pressure 100/60 mm Hg, moderately severe dehydration, and no focal neurologic signs. The patient weighed 60 kg. Pertinent laboratory data are shown below:

2:00 A.M.
Na	140 mEq/L
K	5.6 mEq/L
Cl	105 mEq/L
HCO$_3$	4 mEq/L
pH	6.92
PCO$_2$	14 mm Hg

1. What is the acid-base disturbance? Is the compensation appropriate?
2. What are the possible causes?
3. What other data would you need to determine the cause?
4. Are there any chemistries besides the acid-base variables that should be noted by the clinician in terms of anticipating the patient's course?
5. What therapy does the patient need to receive?
6. How much bicarbonate would you give, and how would you give it?
7. Write your initial intravenous therapy orders.
8. From 2:00 A.M. until 9:00 A.M., the patient received 2,500 ml of saline, 6 ampules of NaHCO$_3$, 150 units of insulin (bolus therapy), and 20 mEq of potassium chloride (KCl). At 9:00 A.M., the following laboratory values were obtained:

Glucose	488 mg/100 ml
HCO$_3$	10 mEq/L
pH	7.05
PCO$_2$	37 mm Hg

What is the acid-base disturbance at this point?
9. What possibilities should be considered for an increase in PCO$_2$ in this setting?
10. What bedside "test" would help delineate the cause?
11. The patient was given 3 additional ampules of NaHCO$_3$ after the physicians received the 9:00 A.M. laboratory values. Is that what you would do?

12. At 10:00 A.M. (1 hour later), the following data were obtained:

Na	154 mEq/L	pH	7.14
K	1.7 mEq/L	PCO$_2$	43 mm Hg
Cl	116 mEq/L	Temperature	39°C
HCO$_3$	12 mEq/L	Blood pressure	70/0 mm Hg

    What problems are revealed in these data? What would you do now?
13. Why is the patient's serum sodium now 154 mEq per liter?
14. In the next 6 hours (10:00 A.M.–4:00 P.M.), the patient received 9 liters of 0.45% saline, 400 mEq of KCl, 350 units of insulin (bolus therapy), and 3 more ampules of NaHCO$_3$.

    At 4:00 P.M., the following data were obtained:

Glucose	690 mg/100 ml	HCO$_3$	18 mEq/L
Na	151 mEq/L	pH	7.37
K	3.5 mEq/L	PCO$_2$	23 mm Hg (on ventilator)
Cl	118 mEq/L		

    The patient's blood pressure was now 110/80 mm Hg. He was beginning to develop diffuse rales and mild hypoxia. Chest x-ray was compatible with early adult respiratory distress syndrome.

    At this time, what would you do in terms of fluid, KCl, and insulin?

Solutions to Specific Patient Problems
Patient A

1. The approach to acid-base disturbance is always the same: If one has data on all the acid-base variables, look first at pH, then at PCO$_2$, HCO$_3$, and anion gap (Δ).

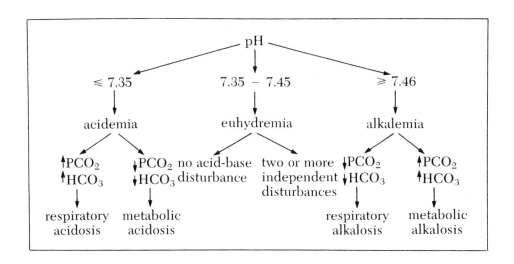

This patient has an acidemia, pH 7.25. Therefore, at least one of her disturbances must be an acidosis. Since the PCO_2 is 14 mm Hg, respiratory acidosis is not the cause of the acidemia. Therefore, metabolic acidosis must be present. The serum bicarbonate concentration of 5 mEq per liter confirms this. The anion gap of 10 mEq per liter is normal; therefore, the patient has a hyperchloremic acidosis. In determining the presence of hyperchloremia, one must consider the chloride in relation to the sodium. In this instance, the sodium is low, and the chloride is above the range of normal and hence compatible with hyperchloremic acidosis.

The PCO_2 is appropriate for the degree of hypobicarbonatemia. The ΔHCO_3 is 20 (25 [normal serum bicarbonate concentration] $- 5 = 20$). Appropriate respiratory compensation is a ΔPCO_2 equal to 1.0 to 1.5 $\times$ ΔHCO_3 or 1.0 to 1.5 $\times$ 20 or 20 to 30 mm Hg decrease in PCO_2. The observed ΔPCO_2 of 26 mm Hg (40 [normal PCO_2] $- 14$) is within this range.

The most likely causes of the acidosis are diarrhea, mild renal disease with aldosterone deficiency in the form of hyporeninemic hypoaldosteronism, or RTA from acetazolamide therapy or perhaps multiple myeloma.

2. Diarrhea is the most common cause of hyperchloremic acidosis. The stool on the patient's clothing, her dehydration, and her low serum potassium (which is lost in the stool) support the diagnosis of diarrhea.

   The elevated BUN and creatinine could be compatible with chronic renal failure (see Chap. 2). Hyporeninemic hypoaldosteronism is associated with moderate impairment of renal function, particularly in diabetic patients. Hyperchloremic acidosis can occur with this and therefore deserves consideration. However, the degree of the hypobicarbonatemia and the low potassium do not support the diagnosis of hyporeninemic hypoaldosteronism (see page 29). The patient could have RTA, which would explain the acidosis and low serum potassium (which is lost in the urine along with bicarbonate). Because sodium is also lost with bicarbonate, patients with RTA are frequently dehydrated. However, the severity of the hypobicarbonatemia would be unusual for either Type I or II RTA.

3. The two most tenable diagnoses are RTA or diarrhea. RTA in an older woman is most likely proximal, secondary to multiple myeloma, amyloid, nephrotic syndrome, or acetazolamide therapy for glaucoma. Acetazolamide also seems to impair distal acidification. Urine pH might be helpful; if the urine pH were greater than 5.4, distal RTA would be suggested, and acetazolamide, which can cause a proximal and distal RTA, could be the culprit.

   Does a urine pH of less than 5.4 exclude RTA as a diagnostic possibility?

No, it does not rule out proximal RTA, since with a bicarbonate concentration of less than 12 mEq per liter one would expect an acidified urine in proximal RTA.

How could one then answer the question of proximal RTA?

As the patient recovers, another urine pH could be obtained. If the patient's urine pH becomes greater than 5.4 when the bicarbonate is still low, for example, at 15 mEq per liter, then most likely the patient has proximal RTA.

4. The patient's total potassium deficit is probably greater than 300 mEq. In some circumstances of acidemia, the serum potassium increases by 0.6 mEq per liter for every 0.1 decrement in the serum pH. This is due to a movement of hydrogen ion into cells and potassium out. Therefore, if this patient had a potassium level of 4.0 mEq per liter and then her pH decreased from 7.43 to 7.27 ($\downarrow 0.16$), her potassium should have increased about 0.9 mEq per liter and should be about 4.9 mEq per liter. However, this patient's potassium is actually low, 2.5 mEq per liter, suggesting a significant total body deficit (>300 mEq). There is no way, however, to calculate the degree of deficit accurately from readily available data.

5. The four diagnostic possibilities for any patient with increased BUN and creatinine are (a) prerenal azotemia, (b) acute renal failure, (c) obstruction, and (d) chronic renal failure.

    It is important to diagnose prerenal azotemia quickly, since a prolonged prerenal state can result in acute renal failure (see Chap. 2).

6. In prerenal azotemia states such as dehydration and congestive heart failure, the urine flow rate is decreased and contact time is increased; back diffusion is increased and urea clearance falls more than creatinine clearance. This could explain the increased BUN/creatinine ratio in this patient (see Chap. 2).

7. Any dehydrated, volume-depleted patient with orthostatic blood pressure changes needs fluid that can be retained in a vascular space. Such fluids include isotonic crystalloid or colloid. Hypotonic fluids are not retained in the vascular space to as great an extent, since the free water distributes as water always does, that is, two-thirds into the intracellular space and only one-third extracellularly. For example, only 80 ml of a liter of 5% dextrose in water (D5W) is retained in the vascular space (only 8% of body water is in this space). In addition, this patient needs potassium and bicarbonate. The constituents of the isotonic fluid should be determined by the patient's acid-base values.

    For example, in this patient normal saline would probably not be the ideal initial solution because the patient has a greater need for bicarbonate than for chloride at this time.

Ringer's lactate is a possibility because lactate can be converted to bicarbonate with a functional liver. Since there is no reason to suspect severe hepatic disease in this patient, this solution might be given.

Colloid alone is not an ideal choice of fluid in a severely volume-depleted patient because such patients already have increased serum proteins, which by their oncotic effect pull fluid from cells. The oncotic effect of the added colloid may worsen this. The ideal initial fluid is isotonic sodium bicarbonate.

8. $NaHCO_3$ should be given to this patient because a serum bicarbonate of 5 mEq per liter provides little buffer reserve. For example, if the patient developed respiratory muscle weakness secondary to decreased potassium and her serum PCO_2 rose to 34 mm Hg, her serum pH would fall acutely to 7.12.

In general, in hyperchloremic acidosis one corrects serum bicarbonate to 15 mEq per liter. The amount of bicarbonate needed to do this is calculated in the following manner:

At a serum bicarbonate concentration of 5 mEq per liter, the distribution space of bicarbonate is approximately 50 percent of total body weight. As the serum bicarbonate concentration falls lower, the apparent distribution space increases to 80 to 100 percent of total body weight, reflecting the depletion of intracellular and extracellular buffers. Since an amount based on 50 percent of total body weight may underestimate the patient's apparent distribution space, there may be a smaller rise in serum bicarbonate than anticipated.

0.5×50 kg = 25 L distribution space

Desired increase in HCO_3 5 mEq/L $\rightarrow$ 15 mEq/L = 10 mEq/L or 250 mEq or approximately 5½ ampules of $NaHCO_3$ (44 mEq per ampule)

Ampules of $NaHCO_3$ can of course be given as "pushes." What is the problem with this?

Ampules of $NaHCO_3$ are very hypertonic (44 mEq of Na/50 ml). This is like 880 mEq per liter of sodium compared to normal saline, which is 150 mEq per liter of sodium. If large numbers of ampules are given, hypertonicity and hypernatremia can result. This is particularly a problem in the pediatric age group.

A more isotonic solution of $NaHCO_3$ can be made by adding 3 ampules of $NaHCO_3$ to a liter of D5W. In this patient, two such liters could be used as the initial 2 liters of fluid given. This would provide volume expansion and correction of serum bicarbonate at the same time.

Why did we decide to correct to only 15 mEq per liter if a normal serum bicarbonate concentration is 25 mEq per liter?

Correction of serum bicarbonate concentration to a normal level results in a paradoxical cerebrospinal fluid (CSF) acidosis.

If HCO_3 is acutely raised to 25 mEq per liter, the PCO_2 will not acutely return to normal due to the fact that the PCO_2 is largely regulated by CSF pH, which will remain low because of the slow rate of diffusion of bicarbonate into the CSF. However, as a result of peripheral chemoreceptors, some changes in PCO_2 will occur. If this patient's bicarbonate were corrected to 25 mEq per liter, the PCO_2 might increase only to 20 mm Hg, and the pH would rise to approximately 7.59.

Analysis of the acid-base disorder at that point would be acute respiratory alkalosis.

The small rise in PCO_2 that occurred in response to an elevation in the serum bicarbonate would be immediately reflected in the CSF since CO_2 is readily diffusible. The CSF bicarbonate concentration would initially remain unchanged, but CSF pH would fall slightly ($\uparrow PCO_2$ with the same $HCO_3 \rightarrow \downarrow$ pH). Therefore, rapid, total correction of serum bicarbonate concentration to normal results in alkalemia in the extracellular fluid and worsening acidosis in the CSF.

9. Potassium should be given to this patient. Her serum potassium is absolutely low and is even lower in relation to her pH (see #4 above). In addition, with correction of the acidemia, the serum potassium may fall even lower.

A safe rate for providing potassium is 10 mEq per hour at a concentration of 40 mEq per liter. Much higher rates can be given but should be reserved for patients with life-threatening complications of hypokalemia, such as respiratory failure, arrhythmias, rhabdomyolysis, or respiratory muscle paralysis (see Chap. 7).

The concentration of potassium chloride (KCl) in the first liter should depend on the rate at which the first liter is given.

The patient was treated with volume expansion, initially as $NaHCO_3$ and then as normal saline. KCl was also given; over 1 week she received 400 mEq of potassium. With this therapy, the patient awakened, electrolytes returned to normal, BUN fell to 10 mg/100 ml, and creatinine fell to 1.2 mg/100 ml. No specific pathologic condition was found for her 1 week of diarrhea, but it was felt to be compatible with a viral gastroenteritis.

Patient B

1. The patient is acidemic; therefore, at least one disturbance is an acidosis. Respiratory acidosis is not present with a PCO_2 of 14 mm Hg. Therefore, the patient must have a metabolic acidosis. The serum bicarbonate concentration of 4 mEq per liter and the anion gap of 31 mEq per liter confirm the presence of an anion gap metabolic acidosis.

The PCO_2 of 14 mm Hg is appropriate compensation for a serum bicarbonate concentration of 4 mEq per liter. The ΔHCO_3 is 19 mEq per liter, and the predicted ΔPCO_2 should be 1.0 to 1.5 × 19 or 19 to 28 with a PCO_2 of between 12 and 21 mm Hg.

2. In a known diabetic, the differential diagnosis of anion gap metabolic acidosis needs to include diabetic ketoacidosis and lactic acidosis; the latter is more frequent in patients with diabetes than in the general population.

   Although we are not told that the patient was an alcoholic, alcoholism is probably the most common cause of acute hemorrhagic pancreatitis, which this patient had in the past. Therefore, one should consider the anion gap acidosis that occurs in the alcoholic patient, including alcoholic ketoacidosis, alcoholic lactic acidosis, methanol intoxication, and ethylene glycol intoxication. Although simple metabolic acidosis is uncommon in pure salicylate intoxication, it needs to be considered, as the patient may have been taking salicylates for abdominal discomfort.

3. In this patient, a serum glucose measurement and Acetest would be most helpful. A salicylate level and calculation of the osmolar gap would also be indicated.

   The serum glucose was 850 mg/100 ml, and the serum Acetest was positive at 1:12, confirming the diagnosis of diabetic ketoacidosis. Alcoholic ketoacidosis is not associated with this degree of hyperglycemia.

4. The patient's serum potassium concentration is 5.6 mEq per liter, which is an essentially normal serum potassium in the face of a pH of 6.92. Using a correction factor of 0.1 pH unit for 0.6 mEq per liter change of potassium, the potassium concentration would fall to 2.6 mEq per liter if the pH were corrected to 7.42. This observation alerts the clinician to the fact that this patient has severe potassium deficiency and is at risk for hypokalemia during therapy.

   As glucose rises in the extracellular fluid, water is pulled from cells, equalizing osmolality on both sides of the cell membrane, thereby reducing the serum sodium concentration in the extracellular fluid. A rough estimation of the decrease in serum sodium due to this effect is 2 mEq per liter for each 100 mg/100 ml increase in the serum glucose. The normal serum sodium concentration with a glucose of 850 mg/100 ml therefore reflects hyperosmolarity. If all other factors remain unchanged, an increase of 700 mg/100 ml in glucose would result in a fall in the serum sodium of about 14 mEq per liter (140 − 14 = 126). This occurs because of the osmolar forces operating across the semipermeable membrane of the cells. Having made this observation, the physician should provide additional free water to prevent a rise in serum sodium to 154 mEq per liter with correction of the hyperglycemia.

5. The patient needs repletion of volume. A patient in diabetic ketoacidosis usually enters the hospital with a 3- to 4-liter saline deficit. This is a result of the antecedent osmotic diuresis. Some diabetics with very high serum glucose may manifest this intravascular space depletion only after insulin therapy has begun. Initially, the elevated blood glucose and the water it obligates are in the intravascular volume. Once insulin is given, glucose moves into cells; water then also moves out of the vascular space, and hypotension occurs.

   The patient needs insulin therapy to stop acid production and to decrease the serum glucose, ending the osmotic diuresis with its accompanying loss of volume and potassium.

   The patient also requires potassium replacement. The average patient in diabetic ketoacidosis requires 150 mEq to correct total body potassium deficiency. This patient, with a normal serum potassium in the face of severe acidemia, will undoubtedly require more.

   The question of whether this patient needs bicarbonate is controversial. There are those who would not give bicarbonate in diabetic ketoacidosis for the following reasons:
   a. Insulin itself stops acid production.
   b. Once production stops, ongoing ketone metabolism generates new bicarbonate, which will correct the acidemia.
   c. Rapid correction of bicarbonate results in worsening of CSF (see Patient A, #8 above).
   d. Patients with diabetic ketoacidosis have decreased 2,3-diphosphoglycerate (2,3-DPG), and this impairs release of oxygen to the tissues. This is counterbalanced by acidemia. Rapid correction of acidemia aggravates this decreased ability for oxygen release, and the resultant tissue hypoxia may contribute to the rare terminal lactic acidosis seen in diabetic ketoacidosis treated with bicarbonate. Slower restoration of the serum bicarbonate concentration with ketoacid metabolism may provide time for 2,3-DPG replacement.

   Alternative arguments are offered by those who do favor $NaHCO_3$ therapy in this setting:
   a. Life-threatening acidemia is present with little buffer reserve with serum bicarbonate of less than 5 mEq per liter, and correction to 8 mEq per liter may not be detrimental.
   b. Although ketoacids will be metabolized to generate bicarbonate and ammonia will be excreted to make new bicarbonate, this will take 18 to 48 hours.
   c. A decrease in CSF pH occurs during recovery from diabetic ketoacidosis without bicarbonate therapy, since bicarbonate is endogenously generated.

6. Unlike hyperchloremic acidosis in which the serum bicarbonate concentration can be corrected to 12 to 15 mEq per liter (see Patient A above), the serum bicarbonate concentration should be raised to only 10 mEq per liter in the setting of increased anion gap and metabolic acidosis. In this latter instance, the anion is "potential" bicarbonate, since metabolism of these excess anions results in the generation of bicarbonate. However, in diabetic ketoacidosis it may be wise to be even less zealous and correct to 8 mEq per liter. Correcting to a serum bicarbonate of 8 mEq per liter provides adequate buffer reserve but helps avoid the problem of overcorrection and too rapid correction.

HCO_3 4 mEq/L → 8 mEq/L = 4 mEq/L

48 L × 4 mEq/L × 192 mEq of HCO_3 or roughly 4 ampules of $NaHCO_3$

Ideally, this would be given as nearly isotonic $NaHCO_3$ solution rather than ampules of $NaHCO_3$, particularly as the patient is already hypertonic.

7. One liter of 0.5% saline with 2 ampules of $NaHCO_3$ added to run in over 20 minutes and a second liter at about 250 to 300 ml per hour.

Two ampules of $NaHCO_3$ in 0.5% saline provides an isotonic solution for volume expansion and $NaHCO_3$ replacement at the same time (see page 34, Specific Patient Problem, #8). One cannot use D5W with 3 ampules of $NaHCO_3$ added because of the patient's hyperglycemia. The lowest tonicity intravenous fluid without glucose that is readily available is 0.45% normal saline; therefore, this would be the intravenous fluid of choice.

Generally in treating diabetic ketoacidosis, potassium is not given in the first liter of fluid. This is because 95 percent of patients with diabetic ketoacidosis present with hyperkalemia. This patient does not have hyperkalemia and is having two other maneuvers performed that will abruptly decrease his serum potassium: the administration of insulin and $NaHCO_3$, both of which drive potassium into cells.

Potassium can be supplied as KCl. However, since it has now been demonstrated that the serum phosphorus decreases during the recovery from diabetic ketoacidosis, 25 to 50 percent of the potassium can be replaced as potassium phosphate. Ten milliequivalents of potassium phosphate could be added to the first bottle and 20 mEq of KCl to the second.

8. The patient is still acidemic, but his HCO_3 is at the level we were aiming to obtain. If all else had remained the same, his pH should have been what?

$$H^+ = 24 \times \frac{PCO_2}{HCO_3}$$

$$H^+ = 24 \times \frac{14}{10}$$

$$H^+ = 34$$

$$pH = 7.47$$

But the patient's pH is 7.05. Why is that? His PCO_2 has increased to 37 mm Hg. Therefore, he now has a metabolic acidosis and a respiratory acidosis. Some people may object to the use of the term *respiratory acidosis* with a normal PCO_2. However, for a serum bicarbonate concentration of 10 mEq per liter, the PCO_2 should be no higher than 25 mm Hg.

$$\Delta HCO_3 = 25 - 10 = 15$$

Compensation = $\Delta PCO_2 = 1.0$ to $1.5 \times \Delta HCO_3$
$\Delta PCO_2 = (1.0$ to $1.5) \times 15 = 15$ to 22
$PCO_2 = 40 - 15 = 25$ mm Hg

Therefore, from an acid-base point of view, this is an inappropriately high PCO_2 and pathophysiologically represents respiratory acidosis because this PCO_2 is higher than it should be for minimum compensation. This rise in PCO_2 is not due to the increase in serum bicarbonate from 4 to 10 mEq per liter.

9. Any time a patient receives large volumes of fluid containing sodium as this patient has (639 mEq of sodium, 2,500 ml of normal saline, and 6 ampules of $NaHCO_3$), the question of pulmonary edema needs to be raised. In addition, an infection may precipitate diabetic ketoacidosis, and it is possible that the patient had a pneumonia that resulted in more edema with hydration. However, at this point the patient's chest was clear by auscultation.

Worsening central nervous system status is an unlikely cause, as most central nervous system catastrophes increase ventilation. In addition, the patient's neurologic status was unchanged.

The patient received only 20 mEq of KCl in the first 7 hours of therapy. He might be hypokalemic. Severe hypokalemia can produce muscle weakness and paralysis that can affect the respiratory muscles, and this needs to be considered in this patient (see Chap. 7).

Severe hypophosphatemia (serum phosphorus of <1 mg/100 ml) can result in muscle weakness and respiratory failure. Although hypophosphatemia this severe is more common in alcoholic ketoacidosis, it can occur in the setting of diabetic ketoacidosis (see Chap. 9).

10. An electrocardiogram (ECG) would be helpful in determining the possible contribution of hypokalemia. U waves on the ECG in the acidotic diabetic would suggest severe hypokalemia. Their absence would not completely rule out the possibility of hypokalemic respiratory muscle weakness. An ECG was not obtained at this time in the patient. Repeat electrolytes were sent.
11. The major cause of the patient's acidemia at this time is his lack of appropriate respiratory compensation, and intubation should be undertaken.
12. The problems revealed here are
    a. Severe hypokalemia. This is life-threatening hypokalemia, and therefore one must use doses and rates of infusions greater than 10 mEq per hour. Forty milliequivalents of KCl could be given in the next hour. Total extracellular fluid potassium is 60 mEq. Therefore, one must monitor the patient very carefully when doses like this are used. ECG chest lead strips (not the monitor strips) should be examined frequently and serum potassium repeated in 1 hour. If the initial ECG has U waves, the loss of the U wave should mark the point where the rate of infusion should be decreased by at least half.
    b. Respiratory acidosis. In light of the rising PCO_2 and severe hypokalemia, the patient should be intubated to avoid a respiratory arrest from complete muscular paralysis. Potassium cannot be given fast enough to prevent this catastrophe.
    c. Sepsis. The patient needs to be examined carefully again for sites of infection: ears, teeth, chest, abdomen, and urine. Urine and sputum (if available) should be gram stained. Blood, sputum, and urine should be cultured. If abdominal examination suggests a pathologic condition, surgeons should see the patient immediately. A lumbar puncture should be performed and smear and culture done. Broad-spectrum antibiotics should be started.
    d. Hypernatremia. The hypernatremia can easily be managed by increasing the patient's free water. It must be kept in mind that he is now febrile and therefore will have an even greater free water loss.
    e. Metabolic acidosis. The anion gap acidosis is not a severe problem requiring therapy.

    At this time the patient was intubated. Urinalysis was sent to the laboratory, which subsequently revealed 50 to 100 white blood cells per high-power field. Urine, sputum, and blood cultures were sent, and potassium replacement was begun.
13. There are a number of reasons for the rising serum sodium concentration:
    a. Insufficient free water replacement in the face of high insensible loss due to hyperventilation and ongoing osmotic diuresis
    b. Administration of 9 ampules of hypertonic $NaHCO_3$
    c. An increase in serum sodium secondary to a decrease in glucose and subsequent water movement into cells

14. Because of the patient's respiratory status, fluid therapy needs to be markedly reduced. One-half normal saline could continue to be used, as a glucose-containing solution should not be started in the face of a rising blood glucose.

    Potassium has been given at the rate of 70 mEq per hour for 6 hours. The serum potassium concentration has risen markedly; the patient is no longer in danger from hypokalemia. Potassium replacement should be reduced to less than 10 mEq per hour at this time; probably 3 to 4 mEq per hour will be sufficient.

    Insulin therapy needs to be continued in an attempt to lower the rising serum glucose.

    The patient continued to get KCl at the rate of 15 mEq per hour. Fluids were reduced, and another 200 units of insulin was given.

At 4:00 A.M., the following ECG strip was obtained.

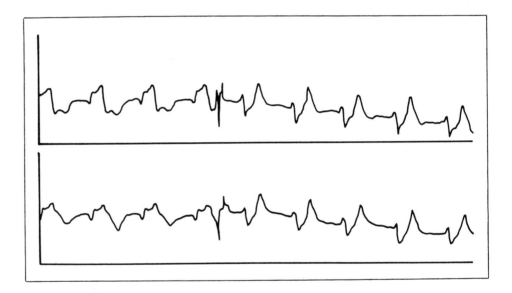

What does this ECG represent?
What would you do at this point?
This ECG is classic for hyperkalemia; there is loss of the P wave, widening of the QRS, and peaked T waves.

At 3:00 A.M., Laboratory data revealed

Glucose	804 mg/100 ml
Na	155 mEq/L
K	9.3 mEq/L
Cl	127 mEq/L
HCO$_3$	9.3 mEq/L

The fastest way to return the ECG to normal is to administer calcium. Calcium directly affects muscular excitability by moving resting potential away from the threshold. It is given as calcium gluconate, 10 to 30 ml. The effect is within 2 to 3 minutes and lasts for about 20 minutes. Once calcium has been given, NaHCO$_3$, insulin, glucose, and

Kayexalate are appropriate therapy for hyperkalemia. As insulin has already been given and glucose is high, these need not be given in this patient. $NaHCO_3$ should be given if the respiratory status permits. As this is an urgent situation, one may have to settle for some transiently increasing pulmonary fluid and hypoxia (providing it is not life-threatening). Dialysis could be instituted shortly if fluid status were such that the sodium load from $NaHCO_3$ could not be tolerated. This patient's chemistries normalized by these maneuvers, but he died of gram-negative septicemia.

Suggested Reading

Emmett, M., and Narins, R. Clinical use of the anion gap. *Medicine* 56:38, 1977.

Kaehny, W. Pathogenesis and Management of Respiratory and Mixed Acid-base Disorders. In R. W. Schrier (Ed.), *Renal and Electrolyte Disorders* (2nd ed.). Boston: Little, Brown, 1978. Pp. 159–181.

Kaehny, W., and Gabow, P. Pathogenesis and Management of Metabolic Acidosis and Alkalosis. In R. W. Schrier (Ed.), *Renal and Electrolyte Disorders* (2nd ed.). Boston: Little, Brown, 1978. Pp. 115–157.

Narins, R., and Goldberg, M. Renal tubular acidosis: Pathophysiology, diagnosis and treatment. *DM* 23(6):1, 1977.

4. Metabolic Alkalosis

General Questions

1. Define *metabolic alkalosis*.
2. Discuss the concept of generation and maintenance in metabolic alkalosis. List the factors that influence tubular bicarbonate (HCO_3) reabsorption, and discuss how these are important in maintenance of metabolic alkalosis.
   Why are the concepts of generation and maintenance relevant to metabolic alkalosis?
3. What are the two major categories of metabolic alkalosis? What is the intravascular volume in these two groups?
4. What laboratory test does one use to place a patient in one of the major categories?
5. If the sodium chloride–responsive group is, in general, the volume-depleted group and the sodium chloride–unresponsive is the euvolemic or even hypervolemic group, why is a spot urine sodium concentration not used in assessing volume as is done in other patients?
6. List the causes of sodium chloride–responsive metabolic alkalosis.
7. List the causes of sodium chloride–unresponsive metabolic alkalosis.
8. Are there some causes of metabolic alkalosis that do not fit into either category?
9. Illustrate with flow diagrams and verbally explain the factors involved in the generation and maintenance of metabolic alkalosis in vomiting, diuretic use, and mineralocorticoid excess.

Solutions to General Questions

1. Metabolic alkalosis is a pathophysiologic process resulting in the loss of hydrogen ion (H^+) or the addition of bicarbonate (HCO_3^-), which if unopposed would result in alkalemia.
2. The pathophysiology of metabolic alkalosis has two aspects: generation and maintenance. It is essential to consider these two aspects, since under "ordinary" circumstances, simply raising the serum bicarbonate concentration, that is, the generation of metabolic alkalosis, does not result in a sustained elevation of the serum bicarbonate concentration. When the serum bicarbonate concentration exceeds 28 mEq per liter, bicarbonate appears in the urine, therefore not allowing for continued increase in serum bicarbonate concentration and returning the serum bicarbonate concentration to 28 mEq per liter. In metabolic alkalosis, some alterations that increase tubular reabsorption of bicarbonate must occur in order to allow the serum bicarbonate concentration to remain above 28 mEq per liter and hence maintain the metabolic alkalosis. The factors are listed below:

Factor	Effect on HCO_3 Reabsorption
↓ extracellular fluid (ECF) volume	↑
↓ potassium (K^+)	↑
↑ PCO_2	↑
↓ parathyroid hormone	↑
↑ distal sodium delivery	↑
↑ mineralocorticoid activity	↑
↑ anion delivery	↑

3. The two major categories of metabolic alkalosis are sodium chloride–responsive (most patients are in this group) and sodium chloride–unresponsive. In general terms, sodium chloride–responsive represents alkalemia with volume depletion, and sodium chloride–unresponsive represents euvolemic alkalemia or alkalemia with volume expansion.
4. A spot urine chloride determination prior to intravenous therapy is the most helpful laboratory test in deciding if a given patient has sodium chloride–responsive or sodium chloride–unresponsive alkalemia.

	Sodium Chloride–Responsive	Sodium Chloride–Unresponsive
Urine chloride concentration	< 10 mEq/L	> 20 mEq/L

However, in many patients, a careful history and physical examination with attention to volume status will be helpful and sufficient.
5. There are a number of factors that influence urine sodium concentration in addition to volume. One of these is anion loss, which obligates cation loss. Specifically, in metabolic alkalosis, bicarbonate can be lost in the urine and a cation must accompany it. Therefore, some sodium is lost as sodium bicarbonate ($NaHCO_3$). However, because the patient is volume depleted and chloride depleted, all the available urine sodium chloride is reabsorbed, and urine chloride concentration is low.
6. Causes of sodium chloride–responsive alkalosis:
   a. Endogenous
      (1) Gastrointestinal loss
         (a) Vomiting (most common)
         (b) Nasogastric tube drainage
         (c) Congenital chloride diarrhea
         (d) Villous adenoma
      (2) Cystic fibrosis
      (3) Rapid correction of chronic hypercapnia

b. Exogenous
   (1) Diuretics
   (2) Plasmanate therapy (acetate)
7. Causes of sodium chloride–unresponsive alkalosis:
   a. Endogenous
      (1) Mineralocorticoid excess
         (a) Primary hyperaldosteronism
         (b) Secondary hyperaldosteronism
         (c) Bartter's syndrome
      (2) Severe K^+ depletion (800–1,000 mEq deficit)
   b. Exogenous—mineralocorticoid excess
      (1) Steroid administration
      (2) Licorice ingestion
8. Miscellaneous causes of metabolic alkalosis:
   a. Bicarbonate ingestion (massive amounts of sodium bicarbonate)
   b. Milk-alkali syndrome
   c. Nonhyperparathyroid hypercalcemia
   d. Carbenicillin or high-dose penicillin therapy
9. The figure below illustrates the factors involved in the generation and maintenance of vomiting-induced metabolic alkalosis.

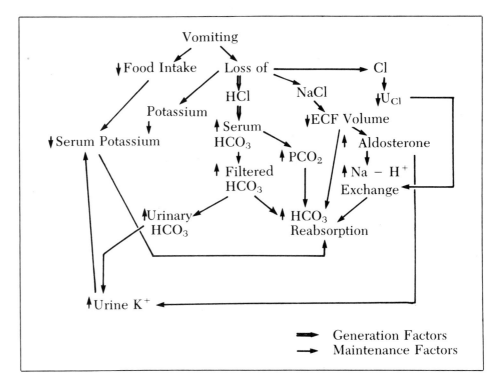

   a. Loss of hydrogen ion can result in the generation of the metabolic alkalosis seen in vomiting.
   b. Chloride (Cl) is lost in the vomitus; this decreases the chloride concentration relative to sodium (Na) in both serum and glomerular filtrate. Therefore, more sodium may be reabsorbed in exchange for hydrogen ion than isoelectrically with chloride.

c. More importantly, sodium chloride (NaCl) is lost, resulting in decreased intravascular volume. A decrease in intravascular volume increases proximal tubular reabsorption of sodium, both as NaCl and as $NaHCO_3$ (Na–H exchange). This later contributes to the maintenance of metabolic alkalosis.
d. Intravascular volume depletion stimulates the renin-angiotensin system. Aldosterone stimulates Na–H and Na–K exchange. The former helps increase bicarbonate reabsorption, maintaining high serum bicarbonate concentration. The increased Na–K exchange is largely responsible for the hypokalemia seen with vomiting.
e. The decreased serum potassium concentration also increases proximal bicarbonate reabsorption, contributing to the maintenance of metabolic alkalosis.
f. An increase in PCO_2 increases bicarbonate reabsorption and is in fact an important determinant of final bicarbonate concentration; that is, failure to raise the PCO_2 in this setting would result in a lower serum bicarbonate concentration than if PCO_2 rose. This happens despite the same losses.

The following figure illustrates factors that are important in the generation and maintenance of diuretic-induced metabolic alkalosis.

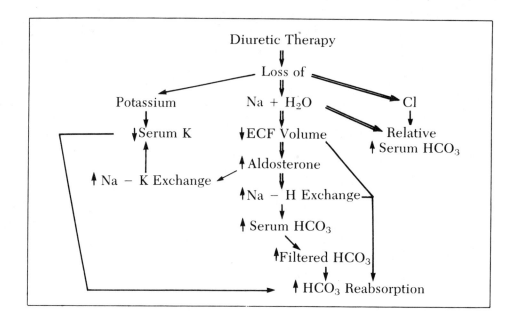

Diuretics block sodium chloride reabsorption in various parts of the nephron. The loss of fluid containing sodium chloride results in intravascular volume depletion, which stimulates the aldosterone secretion; this increases Na–H^+ exchange. The secreted hydrogen ion results in the generation of "new" HCO_3, raising the serum bicarbonate concentration and generating the metabolic alkalosis. Kurtzman [1] gives data showing that in the absence of increased aldosterone levels, the severity of metabolic alkalosis is blunted in diuretic use. Can you think of a clinical example similar to this experiment in which metabolic alkalosis rarely occurs with diuretics despite large sodium chloride losses?*

The generation of metabolic alkalosis as a result of diuretic therapy also is due in part to contraction of the ECF volume. Diuretics cause a loss of NaCl and water, but not bicarbonate. Therefore, the same amount of bicarbonate is now present in a smaller ECF volume, raising the concentration of bicarbonate in the serum. This "contraction alkalosis" is of importance in acute diuresis of large volumes.

In addition, some diuretics, like furosemide, may directly stimulate Na–H$^+$ exchange independent of aldosterone. The increased serum bicarbonate concentration is maintained by decreased serum potassium concentration and ECF volume depletion.

Notice that in this setting the metabolic alkalosis is generated mainly by a factor that in vomiting was only a maintenance factor. Therefore, it is logical to suspect that this would be a milder metabolic alkalosis than that seen with vomiting, and in fact that is generally the case. Serum bicarbonate concentrations greater than 35 to 40 mEq per liter are almost always due to vomiting.

The figure below illustrates the factors involved in mineralocorticoid-related alkalosis.

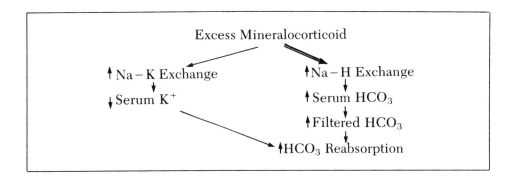

As with diuretics, an increased Na–H exchange generates the metabolic alkalosis. The decreased serum potassium concentration increases proximal tubular reabsorption to maintain the serum bicarbonate concentration. However, as these patients are volume expanded, the increase in ECF volume acts to depress proximal bicarbonate reabsorption. Therefore, this is generally a milder alkalemia than that seen with diuretics. Serum bicarbonate in this setting is usually not greater than 30 mEq per liter.

*Patients with cirrhosis who are treated with spironolactone, which blocks aldosterone's effect, and then furosemide are clinical examples of this.

Specific Patient Problem

A 58-year-old man with a past history of chronic pancreatitis and diabetes was admitted to the hospital with a history of severe vomiting. He had been taking milk and sodium bicarbonate for the associate abdominal pain. On admission, he was semicomatose and very dehydrated, with a blood pressure of 100/60 mm Hg, pulse 120 per minute, with marked orthostatic change in both blood pressure and pulse. No rebound was present on abdominal examination. Stool was negative for blood. The patient weighed 60 kg. Laboratory values were

Na	140 mEq/L	Creatinine	4.6 mg/100 ml
K	3.4 mEq/L	pH	7.86
HCO_3	40 mEq/L	PCO_2	23 mm Hg
Cl	69 mEq/L		

1. What acid-base disturbances are present?
2. What are the life-threatening consequences of a pH in this range?
3. Are any of the laboratory measurements somewhat unusual in light of this pH?
4. What are the possible causes of the increased serum creatinine? How would you evaluate the increased serum creatinine?
5. What are the most likely causes of the metabolic alkalosis in this patient? How would you determine the causes?
6. What are the most likely causes of the metabolic acidosis? How would you assess the metabolic acidosis?
7. List the causes of respiratory alkalosis, and indicate which causes might be operative in this patient.
8. What is the fastest way to alter this or any life-threatening pH?
9. In severe life-threatening alkalemia, what are the treatment options aimed specifically at ameliorating the alkalemia?
10. What therapy does this patient need? What would your initial intravenous therapy orders be?
11. The patient was treated initially with intravenous 0.9% saline. One hour later, the laboratory values were as follows:

Na	142 mEq/L	Cl	69 mEq/L
K	3.5 mEq/L	pH	7.71
HCO_3	47 mEq/L	PCO_2	38 mm Hg

Why did the serum bicarbonate concentration increase? What would you do at this point?

12. The patient was given more normal saline and 20 mEq of 0.1N HCl. Two hours later, the laboratory values were as follows:

Na	148 mEq/L	Cl	74 mEq/L
K	3.8 mEq/L	pH	7.50
HCO_3	41 mEq/L	PCO_2	55 mm Hg

Why is the PCO_2 55 mm Hg? What would you do now?

13. The patient's intravenous fluids were changed from normal saline to ½ normal saline. Twelve hours later, the laboratory values were as follows:

Na	131 mEq/L	Creatinine	2.6 mg/100 ml
K	4.6 mEq/L	pH	7.50
CO_2	33 mEq/L	PCO_2	44 mm Hg
Cl	85 mEq/L		

What does a creatinine of 2.6 mg/100 ml within 18 hours of admission tell you about the cause of the initial increased serum creatinine?

14. Why is the patient hyponatremic?
15. What is the most frequent cause of metabolic alkalosis of this severe degree? Metabolic alkalosis of this severity is usually associated with what other acid-base disturbance?

Solutions to Specific Patient Problem

1. Since the patient is alkalemic, at least one of the acid-base disturbances must be an alkalosis.
    a. Metabolic alkalosis is present. The serum bicarbonate concentration is 40 mEq per liter and could not represent compensation for a PCO_2 of 23 mm Hg. A compensatory response would be a drop in the serum bicarbonate concentration.
    b. Respiratory alkalosis is present. A PCO_2 of 23 mm Hg could not be compensation for an elevated serum bicarbonate concentration of 40 mEq per liter. Compensation would be a rise in PCO_2. Hence, both metabolic and respiratory alkalosis are present.
    c. Metabolic acidosis can be diagnosed from the anion gap of 31 mEq per liter. An increase in the anion gap to 30 mEq per liter or more reflects the occurrence of a common organic acid, such as lactic or keto acid. The low PCO_2 could not be compensation for this metabolic acidosis, as compensatory changes in PCO_2 are determined by the serum bicarbonate concentration, not by the anion gap or the presence of metabolic acidosis per se.
2. A pH in this range represents severe life-threatening alkalemia. The major consequence is cardiac arrhythmias. These can be of any variety and tend to be refractory to therapy.

3. A serum potassium concentration of 3.4 mEq per liter seems slightly high for a pH of 7.86. The predicted change in potassium is 0.6 mEq per liter for each 0.1-unit pH change. Applying that rule to this patient, one finds that if the pH increases 0.4 units, the potassium would decrease by 2.4 mEq per liter: 4.0 (normal potassium concentration) − 2.4 mEq/L = 1.6 mEq/L. Therefore, for a pH of 7.86, 3.4 mEq per liter is a high serum potassium concentration.

   The relative increase in serum potassium concentration in this patient most likely reflects decreased renal excretion as occurs in acute renal failure or increased entry of potassium into the extracellular fluid, as with rhabdomyolysis and release of potassium from muscle stores.
4. An increased serum creatinine in any patient observed for the first time indicates the same four diagnostic possibilities (see Chap. 2).
   a. Prerenal azotemia is compatible with the extreme volume depletion manifested on physical examination.
   b. Acute renal failure needs to be considered in this patient. Prolonged prerenal azotemia or rhabdomyolysis from severe hypokalemia are likely causes.
   c. Chronic renal failure also is possible, perhaps as a part of milk-alkali syndrome in a patient with gastrointestinal complaints, milk and sodium bicarbonate ingestion, and renal failure.
   d. Obstruction secondary to benign prostatic hypertrophy should always be considered as a reason for an elevated creatinine or oliguria in an older man.

   As discussed in Chapter 2, these conditions can be differentiated by utilizing history, past medical records, physical examination, and urinary and serum chemistries: urine sodium, urine osmolality, urine-plasma creatinine ratio, and renal failure index (see Chap. 2). If it is milk-alkali syndrome, renal calcification may be present and may be visualized on an x-ray of the abdomen.
5. Vomiting, sodium bicarbonate ingestion in the face of volume depletion, and the milk-alkali syndrome are the most likely causes of the metabolic alkalosis. A spot urine chloride concentration of less than 20 mEq per liter should be seen in vomiting or in $NaHCO_3$ ingestion in the face of volume depletion.
6. The meaning of an increased anion gap in the face of alkalemia is currently uncertain. Serum proteins, particularly albumin, are the major contributors to normal anion gap. Alkalemia is usually accompanied by volume depletion with a rise in albumin, which then increases its contribution to the anion gap. However, an anion gap greater than 30 mEq per liter reflects a true metabolic acidosis. Therefore, one must consider causes of an anion gap acidosis in this setting.

   Endogenous causes of metabolic acidosis to consider in this patient are
   a. Diabetic ketoacidosis. The patient is a known diabetic.

b. Lactic acidosis, secondary to volume depletion, diabetes, or alcohol.
c. Renal failure. An anion gap of 30 mEq per liter is high for chronic renal failure, but it could be seen in extremely catabolic acute renal failure, such as occurs with rhabdomyolysis.

The exogenous cause of metabolic acidosis to consider is salicylate intoxication, which is consistent with the patient's history of abdominal pain. Most patients in this patient's age range with salicylate intoxication are taking salicylates for pain or other medical problems rather than as a suicide attempt. Also, the combination of an anion gap metabolic acidosis and respiratory alkalosis should always suggest salicylate intoxication, as in adults this is the most common type of acid-base disturbance seen in this setting.

We know that this patient has chronic pancreatitis. Since alcoholism is the most common cause of pancreatitis, the anion gap acidosis seen commonly in alcoholic patients, which includes methanol and ethylene glycol intoxication, should also be considered. However, it is unlikely that either methanol or ethylene glycol would be associated with this extreme alkalemia. As noted in Chapter 3, all these possibilities can be differentiated from one another by serum Acetest measurement, salicylate level, methanol level, and urinalysis, looking for oxalate or hippuric acid crystals and calculation of osmolar gap. Clearly, the Acetest and the salicylate level are statistically more likely to yield helpful data in this particular patient.

7. The causes of respiratory alkalosis are
    a. Pulmonary disease (e.g., pneumonia)
    b. Hypoxia
    c. Central nervous system disease (e.g., tumor, meningitis)
    d. Severe hepatic dysfunction (e.g., cirrhosis)
    e. Shock
    f. Sepsis (may precede other signs)
    g. Pregnancy (easily eliminated in this patient)
    h. Salicylate intoxication
    i. Progesterone therapy
    j. Respirator overventilation
    k. Anxiety (unlikely in a semicomatose patient)

In this patient, the most probable causes of the respiratory alkalosis include hepatic disease (because of the association of pancreatitis and alcoholic liver disease), shock, sepsis, and salicylate intoxication.

8. The fastest way to alter pH in any setting is to alter the PCO_2. In this setting, if the PCO_2 were raised, the pH would fall immediately. For example, for a serum bicarbonate concentration of 40 mEq per liter, the appropriate PCO_2 would be between 48 and 55 mEq per liter:

0.5 to 1.0 × ΔHCO_3

0.5 to 1.0 × (40 mEq/L − 25)

0.5 × 15 = 7.5; PCO_2 = 40 mm Hg + 7.5 mm Hg = 47.5 mm Hg

1 × 15 = 15; PCO_2 = 40 mm Hg + 15 mm Hg = 55 mm Hg

Thus, the PCO_2 should be between 48 and 55 mm Hg. Raising the PCO_2 acutely to 55 mm Hg would yield a pH of 7.5.

$$H^+ = 24 \times \frac{PCO_2}{HCO_3}; H^+ = 24 \times \frac{55}{40}$$

H^+ = 33, or a pH of 7.48

This would take the patient's pH out of the life-threatening range. This increase in PCO_2 could be accomplished by intubation and increasing dead space or by suppressing respiration centrally.

9. The treatment options in severe alkalemia, besides rapid volume expansion with normal saline, are as follows:
   a. Alteration of PCO_2 (see #8 above).
   b. Hydrochloric acid (HCl) is administered in a concentration of 0.15N HCl at a rate that does not exceed 10 mEq per hour. This must be given either in a subclavian or femoral vein to prevent erosion of the vessel wall. Although HCl may seem to be an ideal therapy, the concentration and rate at which it can be administered limit its usefulness as a method for rapid pH correction.

   For example, to correct the bicarbonate excess in this patient would require 450 mEq of hydrogen ion. This is derived in the following way: Bicarbonate distribution space = 50% of total body weight. The patient weighs 60 kg; ΔHCO_3 = 25 − 40 = 15; 0.50 × 60 kg × 15 = 450 mEq. At a rate of 10 mEq per hour, one can see this would be a small dent in the excess bicarbonate.
   c. Ammonium chloride (NH_4Cl) is essentially ammonia (NH_3) and HCl after hepatic metabolism. It can be given in a dose of 0.1 gm per kilogram for one or two doses. Its main advantage over HCl is that it can be given in a peripheral vein. Its disadvantage is that the amounts that can be given safely have not been well established. It has been observed to cause hyperammonemia in patients with liver disease and even in normal persons. The dose recommended would be expected to decrease serum bicarbonate concentration by 3 to 4 mEq per liter. Arginine or lysine monohydrochloride are essentially the same as NH_4Cl in terms of advantages and disadvantages. In addition, arginine monohydrochloride has been reported to cause severe hyperkalemia.

d. Acetazolamide (a carbonic anhydrase inhibitor) causes a proximal and, to a limited extent, distal renal tubular acidosis, resulting in the kidney's excreting $NaHCO_3$ and $KHCO_3$. It is given as 250 mg intravenously; urine pH is followed to document a bicarbonate diuresis (urine pH > 7.0). Acetazolamide causes a marked kaluresis; most patients with severe alkalemia are hypokalemic, and this limits its use. In this patient, the serum potassium is high enough to permit the use of acetazolamide; however, the degree of renal impairment may prevent a response. Acetazolamide can be tried. It could be readministered several times in 24 hours while serum potassium and volume were monitored and replaced as needed.

10. In general terms, the patient needs (a) a lower pH and (b) volume expansion.

    This patient's pH is certainly in the life-threatening range. However, the major life-threatening complication of alkalemia, namely an arrhythmia, is not present in this patient. There are certain risks related to either maneuver for quickly lowering the pH. Morphine might well exaggerate the hypotension. In addition, there is no formula that predicts a given increase in PCO_2 for a given dose of morphine. Intubation is frequently accompanied by arrhythmias; in a patient with an arrhythmagenic factor, alkalemia, such an occurrence may well be more likely. Given the risks, one might elect to proceed with one of the slower acting therapeutic modalities while carefully observing and monitoring the patient.

    Initial intravenous therapy should be 1 liter of normal saline as fast as possible and further normal saline at 300 to 400 ml per hour with careful monitoring of the cardiovascular status (rales, S_3, and orthostatic change in blood pressure, pulse, and neck veins). Potassium should not be added to the initial intravenous solution because of the relatively high potassium for the pH, particularly considering the question of acute renal failure. Potassium should be followed closely. If serum potassium begins to fall and urine output is adequate, then potassium chloride should be added.

11. It must be remembered that in general the organic anions, particularly lactate and keto anions, can be metabolized through the tricarboxylic acid cycle using a hydrogen ion and essentially generating a bicarbonate. Therefore, in an anion gap acidosis, therapy that stops production and permits metabolism to predominate will result in a rise in the serum bicarbonate concentration. Theoretically, it is possible for patients to develop worse alkalemia with the initiation of therapy. Although a rise in bicarbonate concentration is frequently seen, the rise is always small compared to the anion gap, and worsening alkalemia rarely, if ever, occurs. A rise in pH does not occur because in this type of disturbance PCO_2 usually rises with initiation of therapy. Continue the previously outlined therapy.

12. When PCO_2 rises during fluid therapy, the question of pulmonary edema should always be raised, even though respiratory alkalosis is a more frequently observed abnormality. In addition, when hypoventilation occurs in an alcoholic patient after hospital admission, treatment-induced hypokalemia and/or hypophosphatemia and secondary respiratory muscle weakness should always be considered.

    Would a PCO_2 of 58 mm Hg be appropriate for the initial bicarbonate if compensation had occurred? (See calculation in #8 above.) The appropriate PCO_2 was calculated to be 55 mm Hg; 58 mm Hg is reasonably close to that. PCO_2 is largely regulated by cerebrospinal fluid (CSF) hydrogen ion concentration. The movement of bicarbonate into and out of the CSF is a moderately slow process, taking 12 to 24 hours to reach equilibrium. Therefore, this patient's CSF bicarbonate is most likely still 40 mEq per liter. If the other primary cause of the respiratory alkalosis were removed, the PCO_2 should change to a level compatible with the CSF bicarbonate. Since the PCO_2 rose with normal saline, shock was probably the cause of the primary respiratory alkalosis. Now that this other primary stimulus was abolished, appropriate compensation occurred. As long as the patient is not hypoxic, which would indicate a mechanism other than the one outlined above, the patient should just be observed. If the patient were hypoxic, causes of respiratory failure would need to be investigated, since one does hypoventilate to compensate for metabolic alkalosis to the point of hypoxia.

13. This rapid a fall in serum creatinine tells you that at least a component of the rise was due to prerenal azotemia. One cannot say for certain that this was not superimposed on an element of chronic renal failure. It seems possible to convert an oliguric acute renal failure to a nonoliguric renal failure. However, one would not expect a precipitous drop in creatinine in that circumstance.

14. Between the previous set of laboratory values and this set, the patient's intravenous therapy was changed to 0.45% saline. A volume-depleted patient will not dilute his urine and excrete free water; volume will be preserved at the expense of tonicity. Therefore, administration of free water to a volume-depleted patient such as this will result in a decreasing serum sodium concentration when the amount administered exceeds insensible loss and any other free water loss (see Chap. 5).

15. Metabolic alkalosis of this severity is virtually always from vomiting. Gastric outlet obstruction should be suspected with a serum bicarbonate concentration greater than 40 mEq per liter. Patients with this condition are severely alkalemic, since they are gastric hypersecretors and vomit most of their gastric contents. Alkalemia in this range is virtually always due to combined metabolic and respiratory alkalosis. This patient had an ulcer and gastric outlet obstruction.

Reference

Kurtzman, N. A. Pathophysiology of metabolic alkalosis. *Arch. Intern. Med.* 131: 702, 1973.

Suggested Reading

Kaehny, W. D. Pathogenesis and Management of Respiratory and Mixed Acid-Base Disorders. In R. W. Schrier (Ed.), *Renal and Electrolyte Disorders* (2nd ed.). Boston: Little, Brown, 1980. Pp. 159–182.

Kaehny, W. D., and Gabow, P. A. Pathogenesis and Management of Metabolic Acidosis and Alkalosis. In R. W. Schrier (Ed.), *Renal and Electrolyte Disorders* (2nd ed.). Boston: Little, Brown, 1980. Pp. 115–158.

Kurtzman, N. A. Pathophysiology of metabolic alkalosis. *Arch. Intern. Med.* 131:702, 1973.

Seldin, D., and Rector, F. C. The generation and maintenance of metabolic alkalosis. *Kidney Int.* 1:306, 1972.

5. Hyponatremia

General Questions

1. What is the first question you should ask when you see a low serum sodium reported by the laboratory?
2. List the causes of pseudohyponatremia, and explain the mechanism in each.
3. What is the one abnormality that is common to all patients with true hyponatremia?
4. What are the factors involved in the kidney's ability to excrete free water? What common factors interfere with these?
5. Calculate the maximal free water clearance in a normal individual.
6. What is the relationship between the serum sodium concentration and total body sodium?
7. Make a table listing the three major categories of hyponatremia, their causes, and the major physical findings, the factors impairing free water clearance, the urine sodium (U_{Na}), the urine osmolality, and the general aim of treatment in each.
8. List the criteria for the diagnosis of the syndrome of inappropriate antidiuretic hormone secretion (SIADH), and discuss the logic for each of the criteria.
9. List some of the common causes of SIADH.
10. What are the modes of therapy in SIADH? What determines how one treats a given patient?

Solutions to General Questions

1. Is the hyponatremia real? In the acid-base disturbances we have been discussing, there are no pseudo disturbances, that is, a serum bicarbonate concentration of 10 mEq per liter always represents an acid-base disturbance. However, there are causes of a low serum sodium concentration that do not represent hypoosmolality.
2. Pseudohyponatremia does not mean that the measured low serum sodium concentration is incorrect, but rather that the low serum sodium does not necessarily represent a low serum osmolality. The causes of pseudohyponatremia are hyperglycemia, hyperlipidemia, and hyperproteinemia.

    In hyperglycemia, glucose is essentially "trapped" in the extracellular fluid (ECF). Since the ECF and intracellular fluid (ICF) are separated by a semipermeable membrane, water moves to the ECF from the ICF to equalize osmolality on both sides of the membrane. This movement of water dilutes the serum sodium and decreases the measured concentration. The measurement itself is correct, and this is pseudo only in the sense that plasma hypoosmolality need not exist. The serum osmolality cannot be roughly estimated by 2 × serum sodium concentration in this setting. In fact, such a patient may be hyperosmolar with a serum sodium (S_{Na}) of 120 mEq per liter. For example:

S_{Na} = 120 mEq/L

Glucose = 1,000 mg/100 ml

Osmolality = 300 mOsm

A number of correction factors exist for this. A reasonable one is for each 100 mg/100 ml increase in the serum glucose, the serum sodium concentration decreases by 2 mEq per liter. Hyperlipidemia and hyperproteinemia also cause pseudohyponatremia, albeit by a different mechanism. In the determination of the serum sodium concentration, the assumption is made that over 95 percent of the plasma is water and therefore available as a sodium distribution space. This is not the case with extreme elevation of lipids and protein. In that situation, perhaps only 85 percent of a given volume of plasma is water and therefore available as a sodium space. One is then reporting a concentration per liter of plasma, whereas the sodium may be distributed in 850 ml. If one measured sodium concentration in that 850 ml, it would be normal. Hence, osmolality is normal, despite low serum sodium concentration.

The major lipid component that correlates best with the degree of electrolyte changes is the triglycerides. A formula does exist for correcting electrolyte concentrations to the observed changes in triglycerides. However, as triglyceride measurements are not generally rapidly available, a measured osmolality is probably still the most practical way to assess this phenomenon in a hyponatremic patient. Triglyceride-related pseudohyponatremia is not clinically important until triglycerides exceed 1,500 mg/100 ml. The formula is [1]

% increase in electrolytes = 2.1 × triglycerides (gm/100 ml) − 0.6

The hyperproteinemia that produces pseudohyponatremia is not the increase in albumin one sees with dehydration, but rather the marked increase in proteins one sees in such settings as the macroglobulinemias.

There is no correction factor for proteins. Osmolality must be measured.
3. In all true cases of hyponatremia, the kidney is unable to clear free water normally.
4. In order to generate free water, the kidney must deliver adequate amounts of filtrate to distal sites where solute is separated from water. Therefore to achieve this one must have
   a. Adequate glomerular filtration rate (GFR). If GFR is markedly reduced, the total amount of filtrate available to be freed of sodium chloride (NaCl) is reduced.
   b. Adequate distal delivery. In certain clinical settings, such as dehydration and congestive heart failure, proximal tubular reabsorption is increased, and the absolute amount of filtrate delivered distally is reduced.

c. Functioning loop of Henle and cortical diluting sites. These sites must be able to remove NaCl from the filtrate without the concomitant movement of water. Clinically the factors that interfere with this are diuretics. Furosemide and ethacrynic acid block NaCl reabsorption in the loop and thiazides in the cortical diluting sites.
d. The ability to turn off vasopressin (antidiuretic hormone [ADH]). If ADH is circulating in response to some nonosmotic factor, a dilute urine will not be made.
e. Glucocorticoids. These seem to be necessary in order to maximally suppress ADH.
5. If the GFR is 100 ml per minute and 20 percent of the GFR is delivered distally to diluting sites and is therefore potentially available for free water, approximately 28 liters of free water can be excreted per day.

$$100 \text{ ml/min} \times 1{,}440 \text{ min/day} \times 0.20 = 28.8 \text{ L/day}$$

This should make it clear that if free water clearance is normal, it is almost impossible simply to drink oneself into hyponatremia.
6. The serum sodium concentration is merely a concentration term reflecting relationship of total body sodium and total body water (Na/TBW). It tells one nothing about absolute amounts of either.
7. The three major categories of hyponatremia are outlined in the table below.

	With ↓ Total Body Sodium (Na)	With ↑ Total Body Na	With Normal Total Body Na
Causes	1. Gastrointestinal (GI) losses of Na: 　　Vomiting 　　Diarrhea 2. Renal losses: 　　Diuretics 　　Renal tubular acidosis 　　Salt-losing nephropathy 　　Adrenal insufficiency	1. Cardiac failure 2. Hepatic failure 3. Nephrotic syndrome 4. Renal failure	1. Hypothyroidism 2. Glucocorticoid deficiency 3. ↓ total body potassium (K) 4. Inappropriate ADH secretion (SIADH) 5. Drugs 6. ? Reset osmostat 7. Diuretics (occasionally)
Physical findings	Orthostatic hypotension Flat neck veins	Edema Ascites	No orthostatic changes No edema
Mechanism*	Volume depletion: 1. ↓ GFR 1, 2. ↑ proximal reabsorption 1, 2. ↑ ADH	1, 2. Decreased effective volume 3. ↓ volume 1, 2, 4. ↓ GFR (?3), ↓ potential free water filtered 1, 2. ↑ proximal reabsorption	1. ↓ distal delivery 2. ↑ ADH 3. ↑ Na into cells 4. Increase ADH 5. Increase ADH release or sensitivity to present ADH 6. Osmolar sensor changed to perceive low Na as normal 7. Directly inhibits diluting mechanism; ↓ total body K

60 Hyponatremia

	With ↓ Total Body Sodium (Na)	With ↑ Total Body Na	With Normal Total Body Na
Laboratory	GI loss: $U_{Na} < 10$ mEq/L ↑ Urine osmolality Renal loss: $U_{Na} > 20$ mEq/L ↑ Urine osmolality	1, 2, 3. $U_{Na} < 10$ mEq/L ↑ urine osmolality 4. U_{Na} may be >20 mEq/L May be isotonic	$U_{Na} > 20$ mEq/L Urine osmolality >50–70 mOsm
Treatment	Replace volume as normal saline	Restrict NaCl and H_2O or diuretic → loss of NaCl and H_2O; $H_2O > NaCl$	Correct underlying cause; restrict H_2O or ↑ loss of free H_2O.

*Numbers refer to mechanism operative in the cause with the corresponding number.

8. Currently in a clinical setting the diagnosis of SIADH is still a diagnosis of exclusion, and the following criteria have been used to make the diagnosis:
   a. Hyponatremia with hypoosmolality. That is, it cannot be pseudohyponatremia.
   b. Urine osmolality that is not maximally dilute. The urine osmolality does not have to be greater than the plasma osmolality. A patient with a serum sodium concentration of 120 mEq per liter who has a urine osmolality of 150 mOsm has an inappropriately concentrated urine. If urine osmolality were appropriate, it would be 50 to 70 mOsm in the face of hyponatremia.
   c. Normal renal, adrenal, and thyroid function. This is elimination of the other causes of hyponatremia with normal total body sodium.
   d. High urine sodium. Originally this was considered a necessary part of the diagnosis. Generally, urine sodium is high because the patient is on a normal diet and has a low urine volume. For example, a patient eating 80 mEq per day of sodium who has a urine output of 500 ml per day will have a U_{Na} of 160 mEq per liter. However, if the patient is an alcoholic who has been drinking and not eating for 10 days, falls, sustains head trauma, and develops SIADH, he will have a low urine sodium concentration.
   e. Increased serum sodium concentration with water restriction. This is true but in no way distinguishes one type of hyponatremia from another. Since serum sodium is a concentration term, decreasing the amount of water relative to salt will increase serum sodium regardless of the underlying cause.
9. The causes of SIADH are as follows:
   a. Carcinoma
      (1) Lung
      (2) Duodenum
      (3) Pancreas
   b. Pulmonary disorders
      (1) Pneumonia
      (2) Abscess
      (3) Tuberculosis

    c. Central nervous system (CNS) disorders
       (1) Encephalitis
       (2) Meningitis
       (3) Abscess
       (4) Subdural hematoma
       (5) Trauma
       (6) Stroke
       (7) Tumor
       (8) Guillain-Barré syndrome
       (9) Acute intermittent porphyria
      (10) Acute psychosis
    d. Drugs
       (1) Chlorpropamide
       (2) Tolbutamide
       (3) Clofibrate
       (4) Cyclophosphamide
       (5) Morphine
       (6) Barbiturates
       (7) Vincristine
       (8) Nicotine
       (9) Carbamazepine
      (10) Acetaminophen
      (11) Indomethacin
      (12) Isoproterenol

10. The modes of therapy used in SIADH hyponatremia are (a) water restriction, (b) hypertonic saline, and (c) furosemide diuresis with urinary cation and anion replacement.

    Patients with SIADH have normal total body sodium, and their hyponatremia is thus due to water excess. The logic of water restriction is therefore obvious.

    Hypertonic saline was utilized as standard therapy in the past with the intent to raise osmolality acutely. However, what do you think happens when salt is given to an euvolemic or slightly hypervolemic person? The NaCl is promptly excreted, and this is what occurs in these patients. In addition, an elderly patient who is already slightly volume expanded may become markedly hypervolemic and develop acute pulmonary edema in the face of hypertonic saline administration. For these reasons, this method of therapy is now less widely used. However, it will serve to correct serum osmolality acutely.

    Furosemide administration results in the loss of hypotonic fluid (roughly ½ normal saline) that, in itself, would help correct hyponatremia. However, ongoing loss of NaCl would result in decreased total body sodium and volume depletion, and it eventually may perpetuate the hyponatremia. If urine NaCl and potassium chloride (KCl) are replaced milliequivalent for milliequivalent, all the diuresis becomes free water loss, and euvolemia is maintained. This is the current accepted therapy for severe hyponatremia.

The choice of either water restriction or furosemide therapy with loss replacement depends on absolute serum sodium concentration and the clinical condition. A patient with a serum sodium concentration of less than 115 mEq per liter or a patient with neurologic impairment should be rapidly corrected using furosemide and ion replacement. The end point should be a serum sodium of 125 mEq per liter or loss of the neurologic abnormality.

Specific Patient Problems

Patient A

A 60-year-old man was hospitalized because of a persistent cough and 25-pound weight loss over 3 months. He had a 40-pack year smoking history. Chest x-ray showed left pleural effusion. PPD was positive. Physical examination on admission revealed a cachectic man. Vital signs were temperature 37.6°C, pulse 70 per minute, blood pressure 110/70 mm Hg, respiration 18 per minute. There was no orthostatic change in blood pressure or pulse with the patient standing. Neck veins were at the level of the sternal angle at 30 degrees. The findings of the chest examination were compatible with a left pleural effusion. The abdominal examination revealed no masses or organomegaly. There was no edema. The patient weighed 65 kg. The laboratory examination showed

Na	123 mEq/L	Uric acid	3.5 mg/100 ml
K	3.7 mEq/L	Creatinine	0.6 mg/100 ml
Cl	88 mEq/L	Serum osmolality	250 mOsm
Bicarbonate (HCO_3)	24 mEq/L	Urine osmolality	300 mOsm
Blood urea nitrogen (BUN)	4 mg/100 ml	U_{Na}	39 mEq/L

1. What are the causes of hyponatremia that need to be considered in this clinical setting?
2. How do the serum K, HCO_3, BUN, and U_{Na} help in the differential diagnosis of the hyponatremia?
3. To treat this man, should you calculate sodium deficit or water excess?
4. What should your initial treatment be? Write the appropriate initial orders, and justify them.

5. What would be the indications for conservative versus aggressive therapy?

The patient was found to have oat cell carcinoma of the lung. Hyponatremia initially corrected with fluid restriction of 1,000 ml per day. However, the patient could not comply with this, and hyponatremia recurred with a serum sodium of 115 mEq per liter. What would your approach be at this point?

Patient B

N. G. was a 38-year-old man who entered the emergency room with a seizure and a history of 1 week of mental decompensation. On physical examination he was seizing and appeared euvolemic; he had meningeal signs without focal neurologic signs or papilledema. He weighed 70 kg. Laboratory values showed

Na	109 mEq/L	HCO_3	21 mEq/L
K	3.4 mEq/L	Urine osmolality	169 mOsm
Cl	78 mEq/L	U_{Na}	45 mEq/L

Cerebrospinal fluid revealed 40 white blood cells, 80 percent monocytes.

1. What are the possible causes of hyponatremia in this clinical setting?
2. Should you calculate NaCl deficit or water excess? Do the appropriate calculation.
3. How would you treat this patient? Why did you pick that therapy? Write your exact orders, and explain the reason for them.

Solutions to Specific Patient Problems
Patient A

1. In order to rule out pseudohyponatremia, a serum glucose should always be obtained in the initial evaluation of hyponatremia. This patient's glucose was normal. With this clinical history, the two leading diagnoses are either a lung tumor or tuberculosis.

    The mechanisms of hyponatremia in these settings are the following:
    a. Tumor:
        (1) Direct secretion of vasopressin-like substance.
        (2) Metastasis to CNS or adrenal glands: The former causes SIADH and the latter adrenal insufficiency and hyponatremia in the setting of decreased total body sodium. Although lung tumors are the most common tumor to metastasize to the adrenal glands, they rarely cause frank adrenal insufficiency.

b. Tuberculosis:
   (1) Adrenal insufficiency secondary to miliary tuberculosis.
   (2) "Reset osmostat": There is considerable debate among nephrologists as to whether this condition exists. The premise that is made is that in these patients a lower serum sodium is sensed as normal. If patients are returned to a serum sodium of 140 mEq per liter and given a water load, they will retain water until the serum sodium returns to their reset point, behaving as if 140 mEq per liter were hypernatremic; the reverse will also occur. Opponents of this theory see this condition as part of the spectrum of SIADH with a balance between osmotic and nonosmotic factors; that is, the severity of SIADH varies in different patients. In some patients the nonosmotic factors that are responsible for the vasopressin release may be relatively easily blunted or suppressed by the osmotic factor of a lowering of the serum sodium. Hence, certain patients may appear to be "reset" at a level where appropriate osmotic forces suppress the inappropriate nonosmotic forces. This explanation seems to be more in keeping with the physiologic principle of integration of multiple stimuli to produce a given effect.
2. The normal serum potassium and serum bicarbonate and low BUN do not support a diagnosis of adrenal insufficiency secondary to either a tumor or tuberculosis. As these patients lose salt and become volume depleted, BUN should rise. As aldosterone regulates Na–H and Na–K exchange, hydrogen ion and potassium should be retained in aldosterone deficiency, resulting in a hyperchloremic acidosis (HCO_3 approximately 18 mEq/L) and hyperkalemia.

   In SIADH, the patient is slightly volume expanded, and the BUN tends to be low, as does the uric acid (this may be due to increasing urate clearance). Although in SIADH sodium and chloride concentrations fall with the dilution effect, bicarbonate remains within the normal range. From a clinical point of view, it is probably not essential to diagnose a reset osmostat. In this patient, SIADH is the most likely diagnosis.
3. Water excess should be calculated for this patient. This is the pathogenesis of hyponatremia:

   Wt × %water × Na concentration = 140x

   65 kg × 0.6 × 124 = 140x

   $$x = \frac{65 \times 0.6 \times 124}{140}$$

   x = 34.5 L

   Current total body water = 65 × 0.6 = 39 L

   Patient excess H_2O = 39 − 34.5 = 4.5 L

4. In this patient, whose serum sodium concentration is 124 mEq per liter and who is asymptomatic, water restriction is the most appropriate treatment. To correct to 140 mEq per liter, the patient needs to lose 4.5 liters. Let us plan to correct him over 5 days, which would be a 900-ml negative balance per day. How much would you need to restrict him to achieve this?

Insensible loss + urine output − 900 ml = intake

$$\text{Urine output} = \frac{600 \text{ mOsm (required osmolar excretion)}}{300 \text{ mOsm (urine concentration)}}$$

Urine output = 2,000 ml

(800 + 2,000) − 900 = 1,900 ml/day restriction

Thus, a restriction to 1,900 ml per day should result in a 900-ml negative balance per day and correction over 5 days. Of course, the urine osmolality of 300 mOsm may vary, and this may be an overestimate of appropriate intake; therefore, daily electrolytes should be followed. In practice, one generally restricts to about 1,000 ml per day without going through the above calculation.

5. A serum sodium less than 115 mEq per liter and/or altered mental status would require more aggressive therapy.

This patient will likely have SIADH for the remainder of his life, since it is likely the result of production of vasopressin by a tumor. If this were successfully treated with chemotherapy, resolution of SIADH would be expected to occur. However, if the tumor were not treated, one would have to deal with severe hyponatremia on a chronic basis. One could then use a drug that would interfere with the effect of vasopressin on the kidney, resulting in a more dilute urine. Currently the drug of choice is demeclocycline.

Patient B

1. A serum glucose should be obtained to rule out a component of pseudohyponatremia. However, a glucose of 1,600 mg/100 ml would be required to account totally for this degree of hyponatremia.

Change in S_{Na} = 139 − 109 = 30 mEq/L

For each 100 mg/100 ml increase in glucose, Na falls 2 mEq/L

30/2 = 15; 15 × 100 mg/100 ml = the change required

100 mg/100 ml (normal glucose) + 1,500 mg/100 ml = 1,600 mg/100 ml

The serum glucose was not the cause in this patient. This patient appears to fall into the category of euvolemic hyponatremia. This diagnosis is supported by physical examination and urinary sodium concentration. The high U_{Na} could reflect a salt-wasting with volume depletion and subsequent hyponatremia. However, the physical examination is inconsistent with this, as the patient appears euvolemic. Occasionally one sees a patient in whom the initial stimulus for ADH release and water retention is volume depletion who then repletes himself with water, masking the physical examination signs of volume depletion. It seems to be most common with diuretic use and may reflect the other mechanisms of hyponatremia with diuretics: K^+ depletion and direct interference with the diluting mechanism. Therefore, it would be important to know if the patient was taking diuretics or had a history of NaCl losses, such as vomiting within the last 2 weeks. Except for diuretics, however, urine sodium should still be low, even if the physical examination does not clearly reveal volume depletion. If this information were not available, it would be most reasonable to assume euvolemic hyponatremia in light of the physical examination and normal acid-base status (diuretic use, for example, might have shown metabolic alkalosis, with increased bicarbonate).

Given euvolemic hyponatremia in a patient with abnormal cerebrospinal fluid examination, SIADH secondary to meningitis becomes the most likely diagnosis.

2. Calculate water excess.

$70 \text{ kg} \times 0.6 \times 109 = 140x$

$x = 32.7 \text{ L}$

Current total body water = 42 L

$42 - 32.7 = 9.3 \text{ L excess } H_2O$

3. Any patient with hyponatremia and marked CNS abnormality needs immediate correction of the serum sodium in order to establish that this is not the reason for the CNS abnormality. Normally, correction above 125 mEq per liter will improve CNS status. Therefore, recalculate to correct acutely to 125 mEq per liter.

To correct over 5 hours requires about 1,100 ml per hour negative free water balance. Furosemide, 1 mg per kilogram, is given as the initial dose at a rate sufficient to maintain a urine output of about 1,100 ml per hour. The NaCl and KCl lost is replaced as 3% NaCl with added KCl. The first urine after furosemide therapy is sent for measurement of Na, K, and Cl. Before the values are available, one should assume the NaCl concentration in the urine to be about ½ normal saline with about 20 mEq per liter of potassium.

The following calculation is for replacement of urine NaCl loss:

75 mEq/1,000 = x mEq/1,100 ml

x = 82 mEq/L

3% saline = 500 mEq/L or

165 ml = 82 mEq NaCl

One would then follow output in terms of ion loss and replace it hour by hour.

Reference

Steffes, M. W., and Freier, E. F. A simple and precise method of determining true sodium, potassium, and chloride concentrations in hyperlipemia. *J. Lab. Clin. Med.* 88:683, 1976.

Suggested Reading

Hantman, D., et al. Rapid correction of hyponatremia in SIADH. *Ann. Intern. Med.* 78:870, 1973.

Moses, A. M., and Miller, M. Drug-induced dilutional hyponatremia. *N. Engl. J. Med.* 291:1234, 1974.

Schrier, R. W., and Anderson, R. J. Renal Sodium Excretion, Edematous Disorders, and Diuretic Use. In R. W. Schrier (Ed.), *Renal and Electrolyte Disorders* (2nd ed.). Boston: Little, Brown, 1980. Pp. 65–115.

Schrier, R. W., and Berl, T. Disorders of Water Metabolism. In R. W. Schrier (Ed.), *Renal and Electrolyte Disorders* (2nd ed.). Boston: Little, Brown, 1980. Pp. 1–65.

6. Hyperosmolar States

General Questions

1. An absolute or relative increase in which two major substances is responsible for clinical hyperosmolar states?
2. What are the differences between hyperglycemic hyperosmolar nonketotic coma (HHNK) and diabetic ketoacidosis (DKA) in terms of patient age, level of serum glucose, serum osmolality, intravascular volume, serum potassium (K) and bicarbonate (HCO_3) concentration, and aims of therapy?
3. Can you explain why a patient with HHNK who is not in shock on admission can become extremely hypotensive within an hour of initiating therapy?
4. List the general categories and specific causes of hypernatremia.
5. What determines whether a given patient develops hypertonic, isotonic, or hypotonic dehydration?
6. What is the pathophysiologic difference between central and nephrogenic diabetes insipidus (DI)?
7. What are the major causes of nephrogenic DI?
8. How does one differentiate between central DI and nephrogenic DI in a clinical setting?
9. What determines the intial replacement fluid in any patient in a hyperosmolar state?

Solutions to General Questions

1. Glucose and sodium.
2. Comparison of HHNK and DKA:

	HHNK	DKA
Patient age	60	36
Glucose	1,100 mg/100 ml	675 mg/100 ml
Plasma osmolality	380	323
K	5.0 mEq/L	5.3 mEq/L
HCO_3	17 mEq/L	6 mEq/L
Mean fluid required	8 L	6 L

HHNK occurs in an older population, has less acid-base abnormality, and because of the prolonged period of hyperglycemia and osmotic diuresis, has more volume depletion. Some authors have shown a mean fluid replacement of 9 to 10 liters in HHNK.

The major aims of therapy in DKA are to stop acid production by increasing the ability to utilize glucose and to restore electrolyte and volume status. The main aims of therapy in HHNK are to reduce hyperosmolarity and restore volume.

3. In patients with serum glucose in the range of 1,100 mg/100 ml, a large amount of fluid is held in the intravascular space by the osmotic effect of glucose. As insulin is given and glucose moves into cells, fluid follows, markedly decreasing intravascular volume. Rapid lowering of glucose without simultaneous volume replacement can therefore result in hypotension and shock.
4. Hypernatremia can be categorized in a way similar to hyponatremia; that is, hypernatremia with increased, decreased, or normal total body sodium (Na).

Increased Total Body Na	*Decreased Total Body Na*	*Normal Total Body Na*
Hypertonic sodium bicarbonate ($NaHCO_3$)	Gastrointestinal losses Vomiting Diarrhea (usually in children or patients without access to water)	High insensible loss (skin and respiratory)
Hypertonic sodium chloride (NaCl)	Renal loss Osmotic diuresis Diuretics	Diabetes insipidus
NaCl tablets	Excessive sweating	No fluid intake with ongoing normal insensible loss
Substitution of NaCl for sugar in infants' formula		

5. Whether isotonic, hypotonic, or hypertonic dehydration occurs in a patient with loss of NaCl-containing fluid (decreased total body Na) depends on the amount and type of fluid used as replacement. For example, if a patient is vomiting and drinking large quantities of water, he will get hypotonic dehydration; whereas if he has no oral intake, he is likely to develop hypertonic dehydration.
6. With central DI, antidiuretic hormone (ADH) release is abnormal. With nephrogenic DI, circulating ADH fails to cause the appropriate sequence of events at the tubular level to result in increased water permeability of the collecting duct.
7. The major causes of nephrogenic DI are
    a. Chronic renal disease
    b. Metabolic disorder
        (1) Hypokalemia
        (2) Hypercalcemia
        (3) Decreased protein intake

c. Drugs
      (1) Lithium
      (2) Demeclocycline
      (3) Amphotericin
      (4) Methoxyflurane
      (5) Colchicine
      (6) Vinblastine
   d. Systemic diseases
      (1) Sickle cell disease
      (2) Amyloidosis
8. One helpful clinical point in differentiating between central and nephrogenic DI is the severity of concentrating defect. In complete central DI, urine does not reach isotonicity, and urine volumes are high, frequently in excess of 5 to 6 liters per day. In nephrogenic DI, with the exception of congenital DI, urine can be concentrated to isotonicity, and therefore urine output tends to be in the range of 2 liters per day. It follows then that nephrogenic DI is less commonly a cause of clinically important hypertonic states. In a more precise way, central and nephrogenic DI are differentiated by response to vasopressin.

   Sixteen- to 18-hour fluid deprivation is performed in a carefully supervised setting so that no more than 3 to 5 percent of body weight is lost; urine osmolality is then measured. Five units of aqueous vasopressin is then given subcutaneously. Patients with nephrogenic DI should have no increase in urine tonicity with vasopressin, whereas with central DI there is an increase of at least 10 percent after vasopressin administration.

   Other clinical data that may be helpful in differentiating between these conditions are shown below:

	Central DI	Nephrogenic DI
Urine volume	Large	Moderate
Iced/cold preference	++++	±
Onset of polyuria	Sudden	Variable
Nocturia	++++	++

9. Tonicity of initial fluid replacement should depend on the volume status of the patient. A patient with hypernatremia or hyperosmolar coma who has orthostatic hypotension or frank hypotension should receive normal saline to expand volume. In this setting, isotonic fluid is hypotonic to the patient and therefore corrects tonicity and volume simultaneously. Volume is corrected more quickly and tonicity more slowly, which is ideal.

   Colloids are generally not used in this setting because they add to already existing high viscosity and draw fluid from the intracellular space, which is already hypertonic.

Specific Patient Problem

N. L. is an 80-year-old woman who had not been seen by her neighbors for 1 week prior to admission. Finally, the landlord entered her apartment, found her confused and disoriented, and brought her to the emergency room. Prior to this episode, she had been well, caring for herself, and on no medications.

Physical examination revealed a confused, disoriented woman who was markedly dehydrated, with a blood pressure of 80/40 mm Hg and pulse of 110 per minute, with marked orthostatic hypotension. The examination was otherwise unremarkable. The patient's weight was 60 kg.

Laboratory values showed the following:

	Initial	*48 Hours Later*
Na	179 mEq/L	145 mEq/L
K	3.9 mEq/L	4.0 mEq/L
Cl	123 mEq/L	110 mEq/L
HCO_3	22 mEq/L	26 mEq/L
Blood urea nitrogen (BUN)	95 mg/100 ml	45 mg/100 ml
Creatinine	3.1 mg/100 ml	1.6 mg/100 ml
Urine sodium (U_{Na})	8 mEq/L	10 mEq/L
Urine osmolality	738 mOsm	250 mOsm

1. What are the possible causes of the hypernatremia?
2. What is the patient's water deficit?
3. If the patient had merely been in bed without any intake, how long would it have taken her to reach a serum sodium concentration of 179 mEq per liter?
4. Why are the BUN and creatinine increased?
5. What would your initial fluid therapy be?
6. How fast would you aim to correct this deficit? Why?
7. How can cerebral edema occur in this situation if one just replaces the lost water?

Solutions to Specific Patient Problem

1. The causes of hypernatremia to be considered in this setting are (a) nonrenal fluid losses without adequate replacement, and (b) inability of the kidney to conserve water.

Although there is no history of vomiting or diarrhea, the orthostatic hypotension, the marked prerenal azotemia, and the acid-base disturbances (metabolic acidosis and metabolic alkalosis) suggest some nonrenal losses without adequate replacement. An elderly person who lives alone can easily be confined to bed by a viral enteritis, and losses will not be replaced adequately.

In this setting, diabetes insipidus should be entertained also. This diagnosis would not explain the acid-base disorder. Orthostatic hypotension does not usually occur with free water losses unless these are massive. Since only 8 percent of the lost water comes from the intravascular space, a 5-liter loss of water causes a loss of only 400 ml from the intravascular space. Therefore, only with larger water loss will a compromise of the intravascular volume be apparent. However, when serum sodium reaches this level (179 mEq/L), one can see evidence of intravascular volume depletion. A urine osmolality of 738 mOsm essentially rules out nephrogenic or complete central DI; partial DI might be a possibility.

2. The water deficit is calculated as follows:

$$60 \times 0.6 \times 179 = 140x$$

$$x = \frac{60 \times 0.6 \times 179}{140}$$

$$x = 46 \text{ L}$$

$$46 \text{ L} - 36 \text{ L} = 10\text{-L deficit}$$

3. Assuming a urine output of about 800 ml per day (urine osmolality 700 mOsm; obligatory osmolar loss of 500 mOsm) and insensible loss of about 800 ml per day, there would be a 1,600-ml negative balance per day if the patient had no intake.

Deficit 10 L ÷ 1,600 ml/day = 7 days.

This is compatible with her history.

4. As in any dehydrated patient who enters the hospital with increased BUN and creatinine, the choices are prerenal azotemia, acute renal failure, chronic renal failure, or obstruction (see Chap. 2).

The low urine sodium and high urine osmolality are inconsistent with acute renal failure. Given the patient's clinical picture, prerenal azotemia is the most likely diagnosis. The creatinine is increased because volume depletion is sufficiently great to decrease the glomerular filtration rate. The BUN/creatinine ratio is greater than 10 : 1 because urea clearance is flow dependent.

5. The initial intravenous fluid therapy should be normal saline. As mentioned above, only 8 percent of water losses comes from the intravascular space; this distribution of water applies to addition and losses. Therefore, pure water loss ordinarily does not result in orthostatic hypotension. In general, this finding implicates NaCl as well as water loss. In this setting of 10-liter loss, it is possible that the orthostatic hypotension reflects water loss alone. However, one would have to administer water rapidly in large volumes to quickly restore perfusion, and rapid administration is not desirable (see #6 below). One must also remember that normal saline (NaCl 150 mEq/L) is hypotonic relative to this patient's body fluid and will therefore begin to correct tonicity and rapidly restore perfusion. Once intravascular volume is restored, as reflected by an increase in supine blood pressure and a decrease in resting pulse and adequate urine output, one should switch to 5% dextrose in water.
6. Half the 10-liter deficit should be replaced over 24 hours and the remainder corrected over the ensuing 24 to 36 hours. This slow correction has come into common use because of the occurrence of seizures, particularly in children, with rapid correction. The explanation for this seizure activity has been cerebral edema. In terms of osmolality, a decrease of 2 mOsm per hour seems to be an acceptable rate of decline.
7. The following figures help illustrate how cerebral edema can occur in replacing water loss.

```
    A                           B                       C
 ┌────────┐                 ┌────────┐              ┌────────┐
 │  2000  │     − H₂O       │  2000  │   + H₂O      │  2000  │
 │particles│                │particles│             │particles│
 └────────┘                 └────────┘              └────────┘
```

If A is cell size prior to dehydration and B is cell size after, then logically re-addition of H₂O would only return cell size to normal, and cerebral edema should not occur. The explanation for cerebral edema is as follows:

```
                                                         C
    A                           B                   ┌──────────┐
 ┌────────┐                 ┌────────┐              │          │
 │  2000  │     − H₂O       │  3000  │   + H₂O      │   3000   │
 │particles│                │particles│             │ particles│
 └────────┘                 └────────┘              └──────────┘
```

With water loss, there is formation of new intracellular particles or idiogenic osmoles, which protect cell volume. The exact nature of these particles is unclear, but amino acids have been implicated. These generated particles take a finite period of time to return to an osmotically inactive state. In that period of time, the addition of water results in increased cell volume, which in the brain equals cerebral edema with its sequelae.

Suggested Reading

Beigelman, P. M. Severe diabetic ketoacidosis (diabetic coma): 482 episodes in 257 patients; expansive of three years. *Diabetes* 20:490, 1970.

McCurdy, D. K. Hyperosmolar hyperglycemic nonketotic diabetic coma. *Med. Clin. North Am.* 54:683, 1970.

McCurdy, D. K., and Feig, P. U. The hypertonic state. *N. Engl. J. Med.* 297:1444, 1977.

Ross, E. J., and Christie, S. M. Hypernatremia. *Medicine* 48:441, 1969.

Schrier, R. W., and Berl, T. Disorders of Water Metabolism. In R. W. Schrier (Ed.), *Renal and Electrolyte Disorders* (2nd ed.). Boston: Little, Brown, 1980. Pp. 1–64.

7. Disorders of Potassium Metabolism

General Questions

1. What are the major causes of hypokalemia? Explain the pathogenesis of hypokalemia in each instance.
2. Do all hypokalemic states represent potassium-depleted states? Can you give examples in which this is not true? Are there potassium-depleted states in which the serum potassium is normal?
3. How does one differentiate clinically between a renal cause and a nonrenal cause of hypokalemia?
4. Can you estimate the amount of potassium deficit from the serum potassium?
5. What are the sequelae of hypokalemia? Which are life-threatening?
6. What guidelines should you follow in treating hypokalemia?
7. Before one begins an evaluation of hyperkalemia, what question must be asked? How can a partial answer to this question be obtained at the bedside?
8. What are the major regulators of the serum potassium?
9. List the causes of hyperkalemia, and explain the pathogenesis of each.
10. List the sequelae of hyperkalemia that are life-threatening.
11. What determines the need for therapy in a given situation?
12. List the modes of treatment of hyperkalemia, the mechanism of action, the onset and duration of this action, and the limitation of their use.

Solutions to General Questions

1. The causes of hypokalemia can be divided into four major categories:
   a. Redistribution
      (1) Alkalosis
      (2) Familial hypokalemic periodic paralysis
   b. Poor intake
   c. Gastrointestinal losses
      (1) Vomiting, nasogastric suction, etc.
      (2) Diarrhea
      (3) Villous adenoma
      (4) Ureterosigmoidostomy; long or obstructed ureteroileostomy
      (5) Laxative abuse

d. Renal loss
   (1) Osmotic diuresis (glucose)
   (2) Diuretics
   (3) Renal tubular acidosis
   (4) Excess mineralocorticoid effect

   In the redistribution hypokalemia of alkalemia, hydrogen ion (H^+) moves down its concentration gradient out of cells, and potassium (K^+) moves into cells. Estimates have been made that for every increase of 0.1 pH unit, the serum potassium falls by 0.6 mEq per liter.

   Poor intake causes low potassium because it takes the kidney about 2 weeks to adjust to a decreased intake and during that time a negative potassium balance occurs.

   With vomiting, most of the potassium loss is in the urine. Gastric secretion contains only 5 to 10 mEq per liter. The vomiting results in an alkalosis that produces a bicarbonate (HCO_3) diuresis, obligating potassium as the accompanying cation loss (see Chap. 4).

   Lower gastrointestinal losses are a direct loss of potassium in the diarrheal fluid.

   With ureterosigmoidostomies, the colonic segment is presented with sodium chloride (NaCl), which it essentially absorbs in exchange for $KHCO_3$.

   With osmotic diuresis and diuretic therapy, potassium loss largely results from increased flow of sodium-containing fluid. With renal tubular acidosis, increased bicarbonate loss, increased distal flow, and increased aldosterone levels increase potassium loss.

   Mineralocorticoid excess results in increased Na–K exchange. Hypokalemia rarely occurs in secondary hyperaldosterone states until diuretics are administered. Usually, these states have increased proximal reabsorption and decreased delivery of sodium to Na–K exchange sites. Only when diuretics increase distal sodium delivery does frank hypokalemia usually occur.
2. In respiratory alkalosis, in familial hypokalemic periodic paralysis, and in trained runners, hypokalemia is not associated with a deficit of total body potassium. As mentioned above, in the first two instances redistribution is the mechanism of the hypokalemia. The mechanism in athletes is not clear. In uremia, diabetes, and congestive heart failure, total body potassium deficits may be associated with normokalemia or even hyperkalemia.

3. Urine potassium can be of some help in differentiating between gastrointestinal and renal losses as the cause of hypokalemia. If a spot urine potassium is less than 10 mEq per liter, usually this implies a gastrointestinal source of loss and hypokalemia of greater than 2 weeks' duration. If the urine potassium is greater than 20 mEq per liter, this implies either recent onset of hypokalemia and/or a renal site of potassium loss. If one uses a spot urine potassium and a serum pH, one can diagnose the cause of the hypokalemia with a high degree of accuracy.

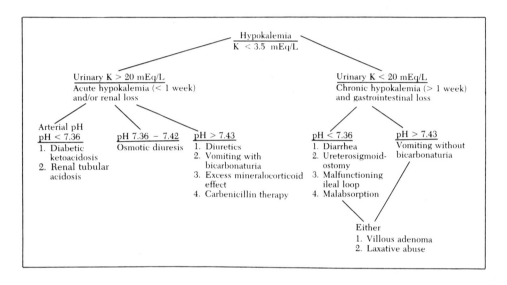

4. Estimations of potassium loss from the serum potassium are poor. Potassium changes related to pH must also be considered. Rough estimates are as follows:

   Potassium decrease from 4 to 3 mEq/L = 150–200 mEq loss

   Potassium decrease from 3 to 2 mEq/L = an additional 200–400 mEq

   Potassium decreased to 1.5 mEq/L or less = 800–1,000 mEq deficit

5. The sequelae of hypokalemia are as follows:
   a. Metabolic and endocrine
      (1) Abnormal glucose tolerance test
      (2) Suppression of insulin release
      (3) Suppression of aldosterone
      (4) Stimulation of glucagon release
   b. Cardiovascular
      (1) Vasoconstriction
      (2) Electrocardiogram (ECG) changes
      (3) Myocardial fibrosis
   c. Neuromuscular
      (1) Ileus
      (2) Weakness; quadriparesis and quadriplegia
      (3) Encephalopathy in patients with liver disease
      (4) Autonomic insufficiency
      (5) Rhabdomyolysis

d. Renal
      (1) Polyuria and polydipsia
      (2) Edema and sodium retention
      (3) Increased ammonia production
      (4) Interstitial nephropathy
   Rhabdomyolysis with consequent hyperkalemic arrhythmias and quadriplegia with respiratory muscle weakness are the life-threatening complications of hypokalemia.
6. In treating a patient with hypokalemia and alkalosis, potassium chloride preparations should be used. In patients with hypokalemia and acidemia, potassium bicarbonate or potassium citrate, gluconate, etc., can be used. If possible, potassium should be replaced orally, as it is considerably more difficult to "overshoot" by that method. If potassium must be given by an intravenous route, the recommended concentration is 40 mEq per liter or less at a rate of 10 mEq per hour or less. If the patient has severe or life-threatening hypokalemia, or if the fluid volume needs to be markedly restricted, both the rate and concentration can be increased. However, in that setting, the ECG and serum potassium must be followed carefully.
7. Before beginning an evaluation of hyperkalemia, one must ask, is this true hyperkalemia or pseudohyperkalemia? An ECG can shed some light on the question. If there are ECG changes of hyperkalemia, then the hyperkalemia is real. If, however, there are no ECG changes of hyperkalemia, it is still possible that true hyperkalemia is present.
8. The major regulators of serum potassium are (a) renal function, (b) aldosterone, (c) insulin, and (d) catecholamines. The first two regulate excretion and the last two regulate intracellular-extracellular potassium distribution.
9. The causes of hyperkalemia are as follows:
   a. Pseudohyperkalemia
      (1) Tourniquet method of drawing blood
      (2) Hemolysis of drawn blood
      (3) Increased white blood cell ($>60,000/mm^3$) or platelet count ($>1,000,000/mm^3$)
   b. True hyperkalemia
      (1) Redistribution
         (a) Acidosis
         (b) Hyperkalemic familial periodic paralysis
         (c) Digitalis intoxication
         (d) Arginine infusions
         (e) β-Adrenergic blockade (possible)
      (2) Decreased excretion
         (a) Chronic or acute renal failure
         (b) Potassium-sparing diuretics
         (c) Deficiency of adrenal steroids—Addison's disease, hyporeninemic hypoaldosteronism
         (d) Selective deficiencies in potassium excretion—systemic lupus erythematosus, sickle cell disease, post-transplantation

(3) Increased input
   (a) Hemolysis, rhabdomyolysis, tumor therapy
   (b) Salt substitutes

In pseudohyperkalemia with increased white blood cells (WBCs) and platelets, these cells release potassium in the clotting process and artificially increase serum potassium. One can avoid this effect by measuring a plasma potassium.

In acidosis, the hydrogen ion moves down its concentration gradient, and potassium moves out, maintaining electrical balance.

In hyperkalemic periodic paralysis, potassium moves out of the muscle under unknown stimulus.

With digitalis intoxication, the membrane pump is impaired, and serum potassium rises. β-Blockade may impair potassium movement into cells by lowering catecholamine-mediated cellular uptake.

The kidney is the main route for potassium excretion, and therefore kidney failure will cause an increase in serum potassium. In chronic renal failure, potassium balance can be maintained on a normal potassium diet until glomerular filtration rate falls below 5 to 10 ml per minute. Potassium-sparing diuretics do not usually result in hyperkalemia unless potassium supplementation is given simultaneously or the patient has renal insufficiency.

As aldosterone is one of the major regulators of potassium secretion, its deficiency decreases potassium secretion. This aldosterone deficiency can reflect total adrenal dysfunction (Addison's disease) or isolated aldosterone deficiency. In adults, this is usually hyporeninemic hypoaldosteronism. This syndrome usually occurs in diabetic patients and patients with interstitial renal disease. The mechanism of the low aldosterone in these patients is not completely defined.

The mechanism of the selective defect in potassium secretion in systemic lupus erythematosus, sickle cell disease, and post-transplantation has not been defined.

Hemolysis, rhabdomyolysis, and tumor cell breakdown during therapy increase potassium by the release of large amounts of cellular potassium into extracellular fluid. Increased exogenous input of potassium does not cause hyperkalemia in a patient with normal renal and adrenal function who is not on potassium-sparing diuretics.

10. The major sequelae of hyperkalemia are neuromuscular and cardiac. The neuromuscular effects are weakness and even paralysis. The cardiac effects include ECG changes: peaked T waves, arrhythmias, and cardiac arrest. The last two and paralysis are life-threatening.

11. The degree of neuromuscular irritability, as reflected by the ECG changes, and the absolute level of serum potassium determine which of these modes of therapy are to be used in a given situation.

With only peaked T waves and/or a serum potassium concentration of about 6.5 mEq per liter, dietary intake needs to be restricted and any potassium-sparing drugs stopped. With more advanced ECG changes or a serum potassium greater than 8 mEq per liter, the first three measures listed in #12 below should be instituted. Dialysis should be instituted when the above measures cannot be utilized or if the hyperkalemia is accompanied by many other fluid and electrolyte abnormalities.

12. The treatment of hyperkalemia is outlined in the table below.

Treatment	Effect	Amount	Onset of Action	Duration of Action	Limitation
Calcium (Ca)	Antagonizes neuromuscular effect	10–30 ml calcium gluconate	2–3 min	20 min	↑ Ca
Insulin & glucose	Redistributes K into cells	10 units insulin 500 ml 10% dextrose in water (D10W)	20 min	2–3 hr	↑ glucose
Sodium bicarbonate	Redistributes K into cells	88 mEq	20 min	2–3 hr	Na load & alkalosis
Kayexalate	Removal of K from body pool	15 gm PO or 50 gm enema	1 hr	Dependent on endogenous input	Na load & requires intact gastrointestinal tract
Peritoneal dialysis	Glucose load HCO$_3$ load Removal of K from body pool			Dependent on endogenous input	Dialysis
Hemodialysis	HCO$_3$ load Removal of K from body			Dependent on endogenous input	Dialysis

Specific Patient Problems

Patient A

K. W. is a 56-year-old, alcoholic man who was found having a seizure on the street and brought into the emergency room. Initial physical examination revealed a man with recurring seizures, blood pressure 110/60 mm Hg, pulse 120 per minute (orthostatic changes were not attempted), respiration 16 per minute and irregular, temperature 38°C, and weight 65 kg. There were no focal neurologic signs or meningeal signs. The remainder of the examination was within normal limits, except for flat neck veins with the patient supine and decreased skin turgor. Examination of cerebrospinal fluid was negative, urinalysis revealed 4+ hemoglobin, 1 to 2 red blood cells (RBCs) per high-power field (HPF), 20 to 40 WBCs per HPF. Initial laboratory data were as follows:

Na	121 mEq/L	pH	7.1	
K	8.9 mEq/L	PCO$_2$	15	mm Hg
HCO$_3$	4.5 mEq/L	Blood urea nitrogen (BUN)	80	mg/100 ml
Cl	77 mEq/L	Glucose	1,415	mg/100 ml

The patient's electrocardiogram is shown below.

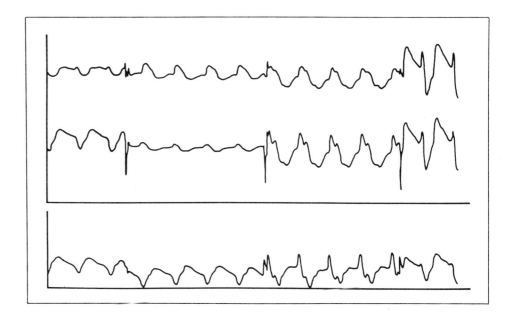

1. Explain each of the abnormal laboratory values this patient had.
2. After seeing this patient and these values, what would you do? List the treatments in order of priority and give your reasons for each.
3. Are there any laboratory tests or maneuvers you would like to do to define clinical problems further?

84 Disorders of Potassium Metabolism

Patient B

S. B. is a 22-year-old woman who is a known solvent sniffer. She came to the emergency room with a 4-day history of increasing fatigue. On the day of admission she experienced pain in her thighs and calves. The pain and weakness increased, and on the evening of admission she was unable to walk. She had one episode of vomiting but denied diarrhea. She was on no medication.

Physical examination on admission revealed blood pressure 140/74 mm Hg, pulse 70 per minute, respiration 20 per minute and deep, temperature 37°C, and weight 45 kg. The remainder of the examination was within normal limits, except for decreased strength in all muscle groups.

Initial laboratory data revealed the following:

Na	140	mEq/L	PCO_2	20	mm Hg
K	2	mEq/L	Urine pH	6.0	
Cl	119	mEq/L	1+ protein		
HCO_3	6	mEq/L	4+ hemoglobin		
BUN	4	mg/100 ml	10 WBCs/HPF		
Creatinine	1.3	mg/100 ml	0–1 RBC/HPF		
pH	7.09				

1. What is this patient's acid-base disturbance?
2. What are the most likely causes of the combination of this acid-base disturbance and the hypokalemia?
3. What additional data would you like?
4. What is the reason for the patient's symptoms?
5. Can you explain the pathogenesis of the orthotolidine-positive urine (dipstick positive for blood)?
6. Why was the BUN 4 mg/100 ml?
7. How would you treat this patient? Would you give potassium? If yes, in what amount, what form, by what route, and at what rate? Would you give bicarbonate therapy? If so, in what form, by what route, and at what rate? Is there any risk in bicarbonate therapy?

Solutions to Specific Patient Problems

Patient A

1. The abnormal laboratory values are as follows:
   a. Decreased serum sodium. There are three possible mechanisms for the observed hyponatremia:
      (1) Pseudohyponatremia secondary to elevated glucose. If glucose were returned to 115 mg/100 ml, a decrease of 1,300 mg/100 ml, the serum sodium concentration would increase by 2 × 13 = 26; 121 + 26 = 147 mEq/L. Actually, this completely explains the low serum sodium.
      (2) However, a volume-depleted patient could be hyponatremic secondary to the volume stimulus to release ADH and retain water.

(3) A patient with recurrent seizures has a central nervous system (CNS) reason for the syndrome of inappropriate antidiuretic hormone secretion (SIADH).

In this patient, neither (2) nor (3) can be considered to be operative, as the change in glucose more than adequately explains the change in serum sodium. In addition, (3) cannot be considered in the face of apparent volume depletion. Although, in fact SIADH may be operative, the patient must be returned to euvolemia before the diagnosis can be established (see Chap. 5).

b. Increased serum potassium. The increase in serum potassium could reflect three separate mechanisms:
   (1) Acidemia with movement of potassium out of cells and hydrogen into cells. The correction factor is a 0.1-unit decrease in pH equals an increase in potassium of 0.6 mEq per liter. A pH of 7.1 is a decrease of 0.3, which would increase serum potassium by 1.8 mEq per liter. Since 8.9 − 1.8 = 7.1 mEq per liter, even after pH correction hyperkalemia persists. In addition, hyperkalemia probably does not occur with lactic acidosis–induced acidemia.
   (2) BUN of 80 mg/100 ml could represent acute renal failure with an increase in serum potassium due to decreased excretion.
   (3) With recurrent seizures, rhabdomyolysis can occur, which can release muscle potassium and may cause hyperkalemia, particularly in the presence of decreased renal function.

c. Serum bicarbonate concentration. A decrease in bicarbonate concentration to this degree can occur only in metabolic acidosis. The anion gap is 41 mEq per liter. The possible causes of the anion gap to be considered in this patient are
   (1) Endogenous:
      (a) Ketoacidosis—diabetic (DKA) or alcoholic (AKA). (Acetest 2 hours after admission was 1 : 8).
      (b) Hyperglycemic hyperosmolar nonketotic coma can be accompanied by severe acidosis, which is not related to ketoacid accumulation.
      (c) Lactic acidosis from seizures.
      (d) Renal failure. Anion gaps of 30 mEq per liter or greater are relatively uncommon from uncomplicated renal failure (see Chap. 3).

(2) Exogenous:
  (a) Ethylene glycol intoxication. The combination of severe acidosis and CNS and renal abnormalities should raise this question.
  (b) Salicylate intoxication. Patients with salicylate intoxication frequently have ketonemia; glucose is usually only mildly elevated. CNS abnormalities are common, particularly if salicylate intoxication is accompanied by acidemia.
  (c) Methanol intoxication should always be considered in an alcoholic patient.
  (d) Paraldehyde causes a pseudoketosis and should be considered in a case of ketonemia and acidemia. This, however, is a very uncommon cause. Large anion gaps of this magnitude are generally due to ketoacidosis, lactic acidosis, or ethylene glycol or methanol intoxication. In this patient, urinary crystals should be looked for and an osmolar gap should be calculated to pursue ethylene glycol; a methanol level should be determined (see Chap. 3).

d. Serum chloride. Chloride will change by the same percentage as does sodium with glucose effect.

$$\frac{26}{121} \text{ as } \frac{x}{77} = \frac{26 \times 77}{121} = 16.5$$

The serum chloride corrected for glucose effect would be 93 mEq per liter. This chloride is slightly low compared to a sodium of 147 mEq per liter. Hypochloremia should always suggest metabolic alkalosis. The presence of metabolic alkalosis is supported by the relationship of Δ anion gap to ΔHCO_3. Ordinarily, in simple metabolic acidosis these are about equal, the fall in the bicarbonate representing the buffering of an equal amount of acid. In this patient, the change in bicarbonate is 20 mEq per liter and the change in Δ anion gap is 30 mEq per liter. The patient, therefore, has a potential HCO_3 of 34 mEq per liter (present HCO_3 + change in anion gap).

e. PCO_2. In compensation for metabolic acidosis, PCO_2 decreases 1.0 to 1.5 mm Hg for each decrease in HCO_3 of 1 mEq per liter. The decrease in HCO_3 is 20 mEq per liter in the patient; therefore, PCO_2 should decrease by 20 to 30 mm Hg. The PCO_2 decreased by 25 mm Hg. Therefore, the patient has simple compensation for metabolic acidosis (see Chap. 3).

f. BUN. This may represent prerenal azotemia secondary to prolonged glucose osmotic diuresis, acute renal failure secondary to dehydration and rhabdomyolysis, or postrenal failure from prostatic enlargement or carcinoma, which is a possibility that must be considered in men in this age group (see Chap. 2).

g. Glucose. Hyperglycemia of this degree usually represents hyperglycemic hyperosmolar nonketotic coma rather than DKA. In this patient, the severe acidosis and ketonemia favor a diagnosis of DKA. However, the patient is obviously hyperosmolar as well (see Chap. 6).

2. In light of the serum potassium and the ECG, the most life-threatening aspect of the patient's illness is the hyperkalemia, and initial efforts should be directed to treating it.

   a. Give calcium gluconate intravenously, 10 ml at first, to be repeated 3 times if necessary, while watching the ECG to see that the QRS complex returns to normal.

   b. NaCl (0.45%) plus 2 ampules of $NaHCO_3$ to run in as fast as possible.

   c. Begin low-dose insulin therapy by infusion. This will treat the increased potassium and the hyperglycemia simultaneously.

   d. Kayexalate enema to remove potassium from the body.

   Next, address the acidosis: Calculate bicarbonate deficit to correct to 8 to 10 mEq per liter.

4 mEq/L − 8 mEq/L = 4 mEq/L

65 kg × 4 mEq/L = 260 mEq or 6 ampules of $NaHCO_3$

Total body weight rather than 50 percent is used as bicarbonate space because intracellular and extracellular buffers are depleted by this degree of acidosis (serum bicarbonate concentration <5 mEq/L). This should be given as isotonic fluid 0.45% NaCl plus 2 ampules of $NaHCO_3$, rather than as $NaHCO_3$ pushes, which are quite hyperosmolar (see Chap. 3). One-half this calculated amount should be given, and the serum pH rechecked.

Next address renal impairment. If the patient were oliguric and did not respond to restoration of euvolemia with adequate urine output, a trial of furosemide and/or mannitol should be given (see Chap. 2).

The patient needs attention to possible infection. Temperature of 38°C (most patients with DKA are mildly hypothermic) and pyuria require culturing, Gram stain of fluids, chest x-ray, and broad-spectrum antibiotic coverage.

88 Disorders of Potassium Metabolism

3. The following additional data need to be obtained:
   a. Serum glutamic oxaloacetic transaminase (SGOT), lactic dehydrogenase (LDH), and creatine phosphokinase (CPK) to document rhabdomyolysis.
   b. Serum calcium and phosphorus to determine possible causes and/or sequelae of rhabdomyolysis. A decrease in serum phosphorus can cause rhabdomyolysis (see Chap. 8). Marked rises in phosphorus can occur from rhabdomyolysis, since it is released from the muscle. This rise in phosphorus can be associated with a marked fall in serum calcium (see Chap. 8).
   c. Serum ketones, salicylate level, alcohol level, and osmolality to aid in defining anion gap acidosis (see Chap. 3).
   d. Plasma creatinine, a spot urine sodium, osmolality, and creatinine to aid in defining the cause of the elevated BUN (see Chap. 2). If glycosuria is present, U_{Na} and RFI are not reliable.

Patient B

1. The patient has a hyperchloremic metabolic acidosis with appropriate respiratory compensation (see Chap. 3).
2. In terms of clinical frequency, the most likely cause of hypokalemia with hyperchloremic acidosis is diarrhea. The patient, however, denied diarrhea. Another possibility is renal tubular acidosis (RTA). The dipstick urine pH of 6.0 in the face of acidemia is suggestive of this. In addition, RTA can occur in solvent sniffers.
3. A spot urine potassium concentration and a urine pH measured by pH meter would be most helpful.
    The urine potassium was 22 mEq per liter, and the urine pH by meter was 6.2, with the systemic pH of 7.09 supporting the diagnosis of distal RTA (see Chap. 3) and renal potassium wasting (see General Questions, above). A component of proximal RTA cannot be excluded. Evidence for proximal tubular dysfunction should be sought. Because of the association of hypokalemia with hypophosphatemia and hypomagnesemia, particularly in the setting of RTA, a serum phosphorus, magnesium, and calcium determination should be obtained.
4. The hypokalemia is sufficiently marked to cause the severe muscle weakness.
5. Orthotolidine-positive urine without red blood cells suggests hemoglobinemia or myoglobinemia (see Chap. 1). The muscle pain and weakness and the association of hypokalemia with rhabdomyolysis make myoglobinemia the more likely of these possibilities. A serum CPK, SGOT, and LDH would be helpful in establishing this diagnosis. In fact, CPK was 1,800 IU, SGOT 850 IU, and LDH 845 IU.
6. A low BUN in a thin substance-abuser usually reflects diminished protein intake.

7. This patient should be given potassium and probably some bicarbonate therapy. Oral potassium may not be advisable, since at this level of serum potassium paralytic ileus may be present. Initial replacement cautiously by intravenous route seems advisable. Because of the coexistence of acidemia, potassium as bicarbonate equivalent, such as potassium acetate, citrate, or gluconate, would be appropriate. However, if these are not readily available in an intravenous form, potassium chloride can be given. If hypophosphatemia is confirmed, potassium phosphate could be given. About 30 mEq of potassium can be given over the first hour as 10 mEq in 100 ml of saline in 3 doses. In between doses, the ECG should be examined for U-wave disappearance (see General Questions, above). Saline is the better choice of vehicle for the potassium than is 5% dextrose in water, as administration of glucose may lower serum potassium by intracellular movement. The RTA associated with solvent abuse is self-limited, lasting only several days after discontinuation of sniffing. Therefore, as in other short-lived acidemias (see Chap. 3, Solutions to Specific Patient Problems, Patient B), there is some controversy about the need for utilizing bicarbonate therapy. In addition, bicarbonate therapy will redistribute potassium into cells and may worsen the hypokalemia acutely if adequate potassium replacement is not occurring concomitantly. However, if potassium is given and bicarbonate is given in amounts sufficient to raise the serum bicarbonate only to 10 mEq per liter, these potential problems should be avoided. The amount needed can be calculated:

45 kg × 0.6 distribution space = 27 L

27(10 − 6) = 108 mEq of $NaHCO_3$

Therefore, 108 mEq of $NaHCO_3$ will be required to raise the serum bicarbonate concentration to 10 mEq per liter. This will radically underestimate the bicarbonate need and produce much less of a rise in serum bicarbonate concentration if a proximal bicarbonate leak is present. This amount of bicarbonate represents about 2½ ampules of $NaHCO_3$ added to 1 liter of ½ normal saline given over 2 hours. This time sequence will permit some potassium replacement.

Suggested Reading

Gabow, P. A., and Peterson, L. N. Disorders of Potassium Metabolism. In R. W. Schrier (Ed.), *Renal and Electrolyte Disorders* (2nd ed.). Boston: Little, Brown, 1980. Pp. 183–222.

Nardone, D. A. Mechanism in hypokalemia: Clinical correlation. *Medicine* 57:435, 1978.

Tannen, R. Disorders of K^+ metabolism. *Kidney Int.* July 1977.

8. Disorders of Calcium Metabolism

General Questions

1. In what states does calcium exist in the serum? What is the physiologically active form? What part of this is measured routinely in the clinical laboratory in the automated chemistry determinations (SMA-12)?
2. What other serum component correlates closely with total serum calcium measurement?
3. What factors are involved in calcium homeostasis? Explain graphically and verbally how calcium homeostasis is accomplished through interaction of these factors and organ function.
4. List the causes of hypercalcemia. Discuss the mechanisms involved in each.
5. Frequently the differential diagnosis of hypercalcemia narrows to hyperparathyroidism or tumor-related hypercalcemia. Therefore, it is worthwhile considering the clinical differences between these conditions. Fill in the following tables.

Clinical Factor	Primary Hyperparathyroidism	Neoplasm
Duration of hypercalcemia (years vs months)		
Duration of symptoms (long vs short)		
Marked weight loss (common vs uncommon)		
Renal calculi (common vs uncommon)		
Peptic ulcer (common vs uncommon)		
Subperiosteal bone resorption on x-ray (may be present vs not present)		
Severe hypercalcemia: serum calcium >14 mg/100 ml (common vs uncommon)		
Serum calcium lowered by steroid therapy (common vs uncommon)		
Serum chloride >102 mEq/L, bicarbonate <23 mEq/L (common vs uncommon)		

6. Are there any physical examination findings that are helpful in assessing the causes of hypercalcemia?
7. What laboratory parameters are used to arrive at a cause for hypercalcemia?
8. What are the symptoms and signs of hypercalcemia?
9. When does hypercalcemia require acute intervention? What modalities of therapy are available? What is the mechanism for the calcium lowering effect, the onset of action, and the potential complications of each therapy?

10. What are the major causes of hypocalcemia? Explain the pathogenesis of the hypocalcemia in each.
11. How does one evaluate a hypocalcemic patient?
12. What are the signs and symptoms of hypocalcemia?
13. What are the indications for therapy for hypocalcemia? How would you treat a patient acutely? Can you calculate a deficit?

Solutions to General Questions

1. Total serum calcium (Ca) is composed of the following:
   a. Protein-bound, 40 percent
   b. Ionized, 55 percent
   c. Complexed, 5 percent

   It is the ionized fraction that is physiologically active. Routine laboratory determination measures the total serum calcium. Diffusible or ionized calcium determinations can be performed by many laboratories if specifically requested.

2. The serum albumin correlates highly with the total serum calcium. The relationship of serum albumin to total serum calcium is closer than the relationship of ionized calcium to total calcium. This reflects the relative constancy of the ionized or physiologically important fraction. The total calcium varies widely, reflecting the marked variations in serum albumin concentrations that occur in a hospitalized population and hence in the protein-bound fraction. It can be estimated that a 1 gm/100 ml change in serum albumin concentration is accompanied by roughly a 1 mg/100 ml change in total serum calcium.

3. The major factors concerned with calcium homeostasis are parathyroid hormone (PTH), vitamin D, and calcitonin. The regulating effects of these hormones are exerted through the gastrointestinal tract, the bones, and the kidneys.

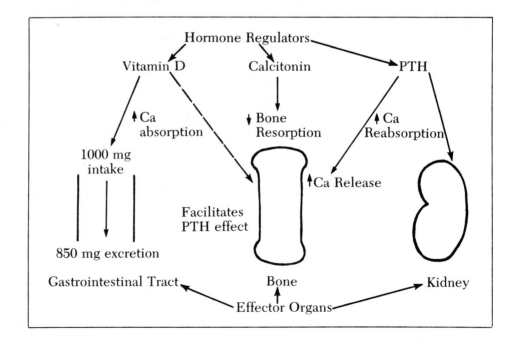

PTH and vitamin D are the major regulators of calcium in humans. PTH is secreted in response to a decrease in serum ionized calcium. Therefore, it is not surprising that the end result of PTH's effects is to increase the serum calcium. This is accomplished through PTH's effect on bone and the kidney. In bone, osteoclastic activity is increased, releasing bone calcium into body fluids. In the kidney, PTH exerts two major effects. One is to increase distal calcium absorption, thereby raising serum calcium concentration. This hormonal effect is mediated by increases in cyclic adenosine monophosphate (cyclic AMP). The other renal effect of PTH is to promote phosphaturia. Indirectly, this may affect the serum calcium in that hypophosphatemia stimulates the conversion of 25-hydroxycholecalciferol ($25(OH)D_3$) into the active metabolite 1,25-dihydroxycholecalciferol ($1,25(OH)_2D_3$). It also seems that PTH enhances vitamin D's effect to stimulate gastrointestinal calcium absorption by increasing formation of $1,25(OH)_2D_3$.

Most vitamin D in humans is endogenously produced. Ultraviolet light exposure converts 7-dihydrocholesterol to cholecalciferol (vitamin D_3). This is further metabolized in the liver to $25(OH)D_3$. In the kidney, this is converted to $1,25(OH)_2D_3$, the active vitamin D metabolite. This conversion is stimulated by PTH and hypophosphatemia. The physiologic function of other vitamin D_3 metabolites, such as $24,25(OH)_2D_3$, is less clear.

Vitamin D stimulates gastrointestinal calcium absorption. This hormone also may promote mineralization of bone matrix and facilitate PTH bone resorption.

Although thyrocalcitonin inhibits bone resorption and may increase bone formation, it seems less important in calcium homeostasis than the other two hormones.

4. The causes of hypercalcemia are as follows:
   a. Neoplasm can cause hypercalcemia by three main mechanisms:
      (1) Metastasis with bone destruction.
      (2) By release of tumor substances like ectopic PTH, vitamin D–like material, and prostaglandins.
      (3) By osteoclastic-activating factors, as in multiple myeloma.
   b. Primary hyperparathyroidism from an adenoma or hyperplasia. Characteristics are discussed in #5 below.
   c. Thiazide diuretics may increase the total serum calcium if intravascular volume depletion occurs with a concomitant increase in the serum albumin. Without this effect, real and sustained hypercalcemia seems to occur in patients with an underlying abnormal PTH axis. The hypercalcemia probably reflects a potentiation of PTH effect.
   d. Sarcoidosis and granulomatous diseases. Hypercalcemia in sarcoidosis results from an increase in circulating $1,25(OH)_2D_3$ and subsequent increased gastrointestinal calcium absorption.

e. Vitamin overdose: hypervitaminosis D (excess vitamin D effect) and hypervitaminosis A. In these times of health food interests and megavitamin therapy, these need to be considered.
f. Milk-alkali syndrome (excess calcium intake) should be considered in the patient with a history of peptic symptoms and heavy milk and antacid intake who presents with hypercalcemia, hyperbicarbonatemia, and renal insufficiency.
g. Endocrine disorders:
   (1) Hyperthyroidism.
   (2) Acromegaly.
   (3) Pheochromocytoma.
   (4) Acute adrenal insufficiency.
   (5) Watery diarrhea, hypokalemia, achlorhydria syndrome.
h. Immobilization in high bone turnover states:
   (1) Paget's disease.
   (2) Metastatic carcinoma.
   (3) Multiple myeloma.
i. Renal disease:
   (1) Diuretic-phase acute renal failure—mobilization of previously deposited calcium.
   (2) Postrenal transplant—increases parathyroid gland mass.
   (3) Chronic renal failure—increases parathyroid gland mass.
j. Phosphate deficiency. The mechanism of the hypercalcemia is not clear.

5. The clinical differences between hyperparathyroidism and tumor-related hypercalcemia are listed in the table below.

Clinical Factor	Primary Hyperparathyroidism	Neoplasm [1]
Duration of hypercalcemia	Years	Months
Duration of symptoms	Long	Short
Marked weight loss	Uncommon	Common
Renal calculi	Common	Uncommon
Peptic ulcer	Common	Uncommon
Subperiosteal bone resorption on x-ray	May be present (not common)	Not present
Severe hypercalcemia: serum calcium >14 mg/100 ml	Uncommon	Common
Serum calcium lowered by steroid therapy	Uncommon	Common
Serum chloride >102 mEq/L, bicarbonate <23 mEq/L	Common	Uncommon

The hyperchloremic acidosis that may occur with hyperparathyroidism reflects the effect of PTH to suppress proximal bicarbonate reabsorption. In tumor-related hypercalcemia secondary to bone metastasis, the serum bicarbonate concentration may even be increased as bone buffers are released and are retained because of the supression of PTH and increased proximal bicarbonate reabsorption.

6. The following physical examination findings are helpful in assessing the causes of hypercalcemia: Hypertension may result from hypercalcemia. Systolic hypertension may suggest hyperthyroidism. Tachycardia could also suggest this diagnosis. Orthostatic hypotension would suggest adrenal insufficiency or pheochromocytoma. Band keratopathy suggests primary hyperparathyroidism. Papilledema can occur with hypervitaminosis A. Parotid enlargement, lymphadenopathy, hepatosplenomegaly, and skin lesion suggest sarcoidosis. Restlessness, sweating, and smooth skin should raise the question of hyperthyroidism.

A good breast examination in a woman and prostatic and testicular examination in a man should be performed, the breast and prostatic examination to assess for the presence of carcinoma and the testicular examination for left varicole, suggesting hypernephroma. Rectal examination and stool guaiac as well as abdominal examination for mass (hypernephroma) are also routine.

7. The following laboratory tests are used to determine the cause of hypercalcemia:
   a. Radiographic techniques such as bone scan, which demonstrates metastatic bone disease, are helpful. Radiographic evidence of hyperparathyroidism such as subperiostial resorption is rare but is helpful if present.
   b. Chloride-phosphate ratio (Cl/PO_4). Since the presence of excess PTH results in an increased excretion of bicarbonate (HCO_3) with a concomitant increase in phosphorus excretion and a decrease in serum phosphorus concentration, it is not surprising that the chloride-phosphorus ratio should be higher (>33) in patients with excess PTH than in patients with hypercalcemia from other causes. Although this is true in many patients, it is not a very sensitive test.
   c. Tubular reabsorption of phosphorus (TRP) is calculated

$$1 - \frac{\text{filtered PO}_4 - \text{excreted PO}_4}{\text{filtered PO}_4}$$

Normal is 82 to 92 percent. This test is performed before and after a calcium infusion. In a normal person, a calcium infusion should result in a TRP greater than 95 percent, reflecting suppression of PTH by calcium and increased phosphorus reabsorption.

d. Serum PTH level. Although measuring the serum PTH level would seem to be the ideal method for confirming hyperparathyroidism and excluding other causes, this has not been true. This probably reflects heterogeneity in circulating forms of PTH, the long half-life of some biologically inactive, immunologic-active fragments, and the "burst" pattern of PTH secretion.
e. Cyclic AMP. As nephrogenous (produced in the kidney) cyclic AMP reflects PTH end-organ effect, it would seem to be discriminatory for high versus normal PTH states. Available data suggest some overlaps. However, the major limitation for clinical usefulness of cyclic AMP is the lack of widespread availability of the test.

8. Virtually all systems are affected by hypercalcemia. The symptoms and signs include
   a. Neurologic and psychiatric
      (1) Depression
      (2) Fatigue
      (3) Malaise
      (4) Confusion, obtundation, coma
      (5) Headache (in crisis)
   b. Musculoskeletal
      (1) Weakness—proximal myopathy in hyperparathyroidism
      (2) Muscle pain
   c. Gastrointestinal
      (1) Anexoria
      (2) Nausea
      (3) Vomiting
      (4) Constipation
      (5) Ulcer disease
   d. Cardiovascular
      (1) Hypertension
      (2) Rarely ventricular tachycardia
      (3) Enhanced digitalis toxicity
   e. Renal
      (1) Polyuria
      (2) Polydipsia
      (3) Nephrolithiasis
      (4) Nephrocalcinosis
   f. Miscellaneous
      (1) Band keratopathy
      (2) Pruritus

9. Hypercalcemia requires immediate treatment in these circumstances:
   a. When central nervous system (CNS) symptoms are present
   b. When the serum level is very high (>13 mg/100 ml)
   c. When the calcium times phosphorus product is greater than 70 to 80

   In assessing the severity of hypercalcemia, it must be related to the serum albumin. For example, a patient with a serum albumin of 1.8 gm/100 ml is markedly hypercalcemic with a serum calcium of 11 mg/100 ml, which would not be the case if the serum albumin were 4.2 gm/100 ml.

   The major therapeutic modalities for hypercalcemia are listed below:

Therapy	Mechanism of Action	Onset of Action	Complications, Limitations
Saline	Increased urinary calcium excretion	4 hr	Volume overload
Furosemide	Increased urinary calcium excretion	4–8 hr	Volume depletion ($\downarrow$ K, $\downarrow$ Mg, $\uparrow$ HCO$_3$)
Corticosteroids	Antagonism of vitamin D effect	(?) 3–6 days	Hypercortisolism
Oral phosphate	Deposition in bone	2–4 days	Diarrhea
Intravenous phosphate	Deposition in bone and in extraskeletal sites	4–8 hr	Extraskeletal calcification
Intravenous sulfate	Increased urinary calcium excretion	4–8 hr	Sodium overload
Mithramycin	PTH or vitamin D antagonism	12–36 hr	Bleeding disorders
EDTA	Sequestered → excretion	15–60 min	Nephrotoxin
Calcitonin	$\downarrow$ bone resorption	6–24 hr	Nausea and vomiting, tachyphylaxis
Dialysis	Removal from body pool	4–8 hr	Complications of dialysis

   The safest and most widely employed acute therapy is saline- and furosemide-induced calciuresis. Five to 6 liters of urine output per day is necessary for effective therapy; euvolemia must be maintained by saline replacement.

   The role of indomethacin, propranolol, and cimetidine in chronic treatment of hypercalcemia remains to be elucidated.

10. The causes of hypocalcemia include
    a. Hypoalbuminemia (pseudohypocalcemia). Total serum calcium will be decreased, but the physiologically active fraction, ionized calcium, will be normal.
    b. Hypomagnesemia. The hypocalcemia associated with hypomagnesemia results from decreased release of PTH as well as some end-organ resistance to the circulating PTH.
    c. Vitamin D deficiency—nutritional, malabsorption, and abnormal metabolism of vitamin D. The last occurs with very severe hepatic insufficiency with failure of $25(OH)D_3$ synthesis; with renal insufficiency with decreased synthesis of $1,25(OH)_2D_3$; and with chronic therapy with anticonvulsants such as Dilantin and phenobarbital. In the last circumstance, hepatic microsomal enzyme activity is increased, and thereby there is increased formation of inactive vitamin D metabolites.
    d. PTH deficiency. The most common cause of hypoparathyroidism is surgical removal of the parathyroid glands, which can occur inadvertently during surgical total thyroidectomy. Rarely, PTH deficiency can result from parathyroid gland irradiation, neoplastic infiltration of the gland, or hemochromatosis involving the gland.
       Genetic hypoparathyroidism can occur alone or in association with multiple end-organ deficiency (e.g., MEDAC, multiple endocrine deficiency, autoimmune candidiasis).
       As stated above, hypomagnesemia can be a cause of PTH deficiency.
    e. Lack of PTH responsiveness—pseudohypoparathyroidism. In these disorders (type 1 and type 2), circulating or exogenous PTH fails to result in an appropriate calcemic response.
    f. Rapid calcium deposition—rhabdomyolysis and acute pancreatitis.
    g. Miscellaneous—osteoblastic tumors (prostate and breast are most common). Although these tumors are frequently associated with hypercalcemia, hypocalcemia can occur. The mechanism is not clear.
    h. Excess calcitonin—medullary carcinoma of the thyroid. This association is surprisingly rare.

11. The evaluation of hypocalcemia might proceed as follows:

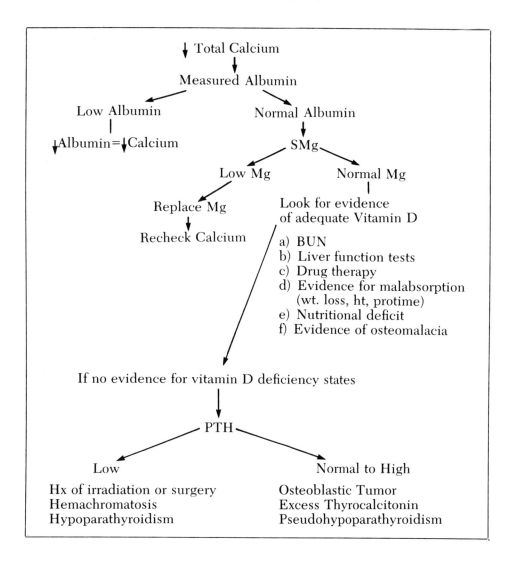

12. The signs and symptoms of hypocalcemia include
    a. Neurologic effects:
       (1) Tetany.
       (2) Spontaneous carpal pedal spasm, laryngeal spasm.
       (3) Latent tetany.
           (a) Chvostek's sign is twitching of the muscles innervated by the facial nerve. It is elicited by gently tapping the cheek about 2 cm anterior to the earlobe, below the zygomatic process.

(b) Trousseau's sign is carpal spasm produced after 2 to 3 minutes of hand ischemia induced by inflating a sphygmomanometer cuff above the patient's systolic blood pressure.
(4) Convulsions.
(5) Mild papilledema
(6) Basal ganglia calcification in hypoparathyroidism.
b. Cardiac effects:
(1) Prolonged Q–T interval.
(2) Refractiveness to digitalis in atrial fibrillation.
(3) Congestive heart failure. Low cardiac output has been reported in acute severe hypocalcemia.
c. Psychiatric effects: Psychoses have been reported.
d. Ectodermal effects:
(1) Brittle nails.
(2) Coarse hair.
(3) Lenticular cataracts.
13. The urgency for therapy and the nature of the therapy depend on the chronicity of the hypocalcemia as well as its cause.

In acute hypocalcemia with evidence of tetany, replacement therapy with calcium salts should be started immediately. If the patient is an alcoholic, magnesium should be administered concomitant with calcium therapy. If there is evidence for rhabdomyolysis, if hyperphosphatemia is known to be present, or if the patient is receiving digitalis, caution should be exercised in giving parenteral calcium. Ten to 20 ml of 10% calcium gluconate can be given as a slow, intravenous "push." If symptoms recur or if calcium remains very low, continuous intravenous infusion should be given as 10 mEq of 10% calcium gluconate in 500 ml of 5% dextrose in water (D5W) over 4 to 6 hours. If the patient can take oral medication, calcium by mouth should also be instituted.

The treatment of chronic hypocalcemia centers around its cause and removal or correction of the pathogenetic factor or factors. A deficit cannot be calculated for this ion.

Specific Patient Problems
Patient A

G. B. is a 75-year-old woman who was brought to the emergency room by her family for increasing confusion. For the last 4 to 5 days she had experienced nausea, vomiting, and constipation. Pertinent past history included subtotal thyroidectomy with subsequent hypoparathyroidism. Her current medicine included vitamin D, 50,000 units daily; calcium lactate, 2,400 mg daily; Synthroid, 200 µg daily; hydrochlorothiazide, 50 mg twice a day; and Klor, 20 mEq twice a day. Physical examination revealed the following: a very lethargic woman; blood pressure 130/76 mm Hg, pulse 70 per minute (lying) and irregularly irregular; blood pressure 110/60 mm Hg, pulse 82 per minute (sitting); temperature 37°C. The remainder of the examination was within normal limits.

Laboratory

Hematocrit (HCT)	33%	BUN	44 mg/100 ml
Na	139 mEq/L	Creatinine	2.2 mEq/L
K	3.4 mEq/L	Uric acid	14 mg/100 ml
Cl	93 mEq/L	Ca	16 mg/100 ml
HCO_3	30 mEq/L	Albumin	4.4 gm/100 ml

1. What factors may be important in causing this patient's hypercalcemia?
2. Which of the patient's symptoms can be explained by the hypercalcemia?
3. What would you do to help diagnose the specific cause of the hypercalcemia?
4. What would you do therapeutically?
5. Can you explain the elevated BUN, creatinine, and uric acid?

Patient B

J. H. is a 25-year-old man who entered the emergency room with complaints of nausea and vomiting of 1 week's duration and pedal edema of 6 to 8 month's duration. His only other pertinent history was of Bright's disease with proteinuria at the age of 7. He had been told several years ago that he had hypertension, but this was not treated. Physical examination revealed a sallow-looking white man. Fundi: A-V nicking; neck veins were 3 cm above the clavicle at 30 degrees. Chest: bibasilar rales; dullness at bases. Heart; S_4 and S_3 without murmurs or rubs. Abdomen: probably minimal ascites. Stool: guaiac negative. Extremities: 3+ edema to thighs. Neurologic: patient somewhat lethargic; 2+ asterixis without focal signs; decreased position and vibratory sense in lower extremities. Urinalysis: 4+ protein; occasional red blood cell and hyaline cast.

Laboratory

HCT	25%	BUN	168 mg/100 ml
White blood cells	5,000	Creatinine	16 mg/100 ml
Na	135 mEq/L	Ca	6 mg/100 ml
K	5.6 mEq/L	PO_4	7.8 mg/100 ml
Cl	100 mEq/L	Albumin	3 gm/100 ml
HCO_3	10 mEq/L		

1. What factors are involved in producing the hypocalcemia in this patient?
2. Would you treat the hypocalcemia? If so, what would you do therapeutically? Would you give calcium?
3. What is the most likely cause of the renal failure?
4. Can you explain the hyperkalemia, low bicarbonate concentration, and elevated serum phosphorus?

A Foley catheter was placed with only 60 ml in the bladder. Two hundred milligrams of furosemide was given. The housestaff was concerned about the hyperkalemia and the low bicarbonate concentration and gave 3 ampules of $NaHCO_3$ as a push and 3 more ampules in 1 liter of D5W to run in over 2 hours. During the infusion the patient developed spontaneous carpal pedal spasm.

What was the reason for this?

Solutions to Specific Patient Problems
Patient A

1. The patient was receiving vitamin D and therefore could have vitamin D intoxication. Although the oral calcium supplement alone would be unlikely to cause hypercalcemia to this degree, the resultant high calcium intake would aggravate vitamin D intoxication by making more calcium available for absorption. The patient also was receiving Synthroid in a somewhat high dose for an elderly woman. This dose plus the presence of atrial fibrillation raises the question of hyperthyroidism. Hyperthyroidism also can cause hypercalcemia, although again rarely to this degree. Hydrochlorothiazide administration is also associated with mild hypercalcemia. All these factors may be contributing to this woman's hypercalcemia. In addition, as severe hypercalcemia is most commonly associated with malignancy, the question of occult malignancy must be entertained.

2. This patient's confusion, nausea, vomiting, and constipation could all be manifestations of her hypercalcemic state.

3. Ideally, one would like to measure a vitamin D level in this patient, but these measurements are not readily available. The role of hyperthyroidism can be evaluated by measurement of triiodothyronine (T_3) and thyroxine (T_4). If these are borderline high, one could most accurately assess exogenous thyroid excess by TRH test, which involves infusing thyrotropin releasing hormone (TRH) and measuring thyroid-stimulating hormone (TSH) response. A measurement of PTH would be of interest, as one would expect this to be unmeasurable in light of the history and the presence of hypercalcemia of this degree. The question of malignancy-related hypercalcemia is less readily evaluated. Initially, a good breast and rectal examination, stool guaiac, chest x-ray, and serum protein electrophoresis (as a screen for multiple myeloma) would be adequate.

4. The patient should be vigorously treated. Initially, the vitamin D, calcium lactate, Synthroid, and hydrochlorothiazide should be discontinued. This is not sufficient therapy, however, particularly since the vitamin D effect might last for weeks to months. The most commonly used therapy is forced saline diuresis mediated by furosemide. Care must be taken to keep the patient euvolemic. In an elderly patient, one also must be aware of the potential for volume overload. However, it is better to err on the side of slight overexpansion rather than dehydration in this setting. Normal saline at 200 to 400 ml per hour should be given intravenously and the patient monitored carefully. Once the patient is euvolemic, without orthostatic hypotension, 40 mg of Lasix should be given intravenously. A urine output of 5 to 6 liters per day should be achieved. One might consider prednisone therapy to blunt gastrointestinal absorption and in that way counteract the vitamin D effect.

104 Disorders of Calcium Metabolism

5. The elevated BUN, creatinine, and uric acid most likely reflect prerenal azotemia from intravascular volume depletion. This volume depletion could have resulted from the hypercalcemia-induced anorexia, decreased intake from confusion, vomiting, and nephrogenic diabetes insipidus. A spot urine sodium concentration and a calculated renal failure index would be helpful in confirming this diagnosis (see Chap. 2). Elevated uric acid with hypercalcemia should always raise the question of rapid cell turnover with malignancy such as occurs in multiple myeloma.

Patient B

1. The first question to ask in relation to hypocalcemia is the level of the serum albumin. One would expect hypoalbuminemia in a patient with 4+ proteinuria. The serum albumin would need to be 1.5 gm/100 ml to explain this degree of hypocalcemia: Calcium is decreased from a low normal of $8.5 - 6.0 = 2.5$ mg/100 ml. This would require a decrease in albumin of roughly the same amount: $4.0 - 2.5 = 1.5$ gm/100 ml. In a somewhat different approach, a normal serum albumin concentration of 4 gm/100 ml would only return the total serum calcium to 7 gm/100 ml. Therefore, another explanation is necessary. This degree of renal insufficiency is often accompanied by hypocalcemia (see General Questions, above).
2. The best initial approach to hypocalcemia in a hyperphosphatemic patient with renal failure is to lower the serum phosphorus content with phosphate binding agents. Calcium supplementation, either orally or intravenously, would not be given until after serum phosphorus has been normalized. Raising the calcium without decreasing the phosphorus concentration would result in an increase in the calcium-phosphorus product and increase the likelihood of soft tissue calcification.
3. The differential diagnosis of an elevated BUN and creatinine in a patient not previously under one's care should include acute renal failure, prerenal azotemia, obstruction, and chronic renal failure (see Chap. 2). The history of previous renal disease (Bright's disease—proteinuria and renal insufficiency), previously noted hypertension, and peripheral neuropathy suggest chronic renal disease. The relative lack of CNS symptomatology in the presence of severe azotemia also suggests a chronic situation. The absolute values of BUN, creatinine, hematocrit, calcium, and phosphate do not differentiate acute from chronic renal failure. The presence of proteinuria and hypoalbuminemia suggest glomerular pathology and make primary obstructive uropathy less likely. The absence of other systemic abnormalities historically or on physical examination suggests a primary renal disease. Considering these factors, the most likely diagnosis is chronic glomerulonephritis. The long history suggests membranous glomerulonephritis.

4. The hyperkalemia is most likely due to renal insufficiency and perhaps to some extent the acidemia. The low bicarbonate concentration and the increased anion gap (25 mEq/L) suggest an anion gap type of metabolic acidosis. This would then be compatible with end-stage renal failure. The hyperphosphatemia reflects the kidney's markedly decreased ability to excrete phosphorus normally.

   The development of carpal pedal spasm most likely reflects the decrease in ionized calcium secondary to the decrease in hydrogen ion concentration after $NaHCO_3$ therapy. $NaHCO_3$ therapy was stopped and the patient carefully monitored.

Reference

Miller, P. D. Diagnosis and treatment of hypercalcemia. Presented at the Kidney Disease and Renal Failure Symposium, Aspen, Colorado, July 8, 1978.

Suggested Reading

Hearsh, H., et al. Primary hyperparathyroidism: Incidence, mobility and potential economic impact in a community. *N. Engl. J. Med.* 302:189, 1980.

Parfitt, A. M., and Kleereker, M. Clinical Disorders of Calcium, Phosphorus and Magnesium Metabolism. In M. H. Maxwell and C. R. Kleeman (Eds.), *Clinical Disorders of Fluid and Electrolyte Metabolism* (3rd ed.). New York: McGraw-Hill, 1980.

Popovtzer, M., and Knochel, J. Disorders of Calcium, Phosphorus, Vitamin D, and Parathyroid Hormone Activity. In R. W. Schrier (Ed.), *Renal and Electrolyte Disorders* (2nd ed.). Boston: Little, Brown, 1980. Pp. 223–298.

Suki, W. W., et al. Acute treatment of hypercalcemia with furosemide. *N. Engl. J. Med.* 283:836, 1970.

9. Disorders of Phosphorus Metabolism

General Questions

1. What factors regulate phosphorus homeostasis?
2. What conditions are associated with severe acute hypophosphatemia, and what is the pathophysiologic mechanism responsible for the hypophosphatemia in each?
3. What other electrolyte abnormalities are frequently associated with severe hypophosphatemia?
4. What are the clinical consequences of severe hypophosphatemia?
5. What are the general therapeutic modalities for severe acute hypophosphatemia?
6. What is the difference between hypophosphatemia and phosphate deficiency? What are the clinical conditions associated with chronic phosphorus deficiency?
7. What are the clinical sequelae of chronic phosphorus deficiency?
8. What are the therapeutic modalities for chronic phosphorus deficiency?
9. List the causes of hyperphosphatemia, and discuss the mechanism involved in each.
10. Which of these causes are the most common?
11. What factors should be considered in deciding to institute therapy?
12. What modalities can be employed to treat hyperphosphatemia?

Solutions to General Questions

1. As with potassium, which is primarily an intracellular ion, serum phosphorus is controlled not only by factors that regulate net absorption (intake absorbed − excretion), but also by factors that regulate intracellular-extracellular distribution.

   The regulator of gastrointestinal absorption is 1,25-dihydroxycholecalciferol ($1,25(OH)_2D_3$). Regulators of excretion are (a) phosphorus intake, (b) parathyroid hormone, (c) intravascular volume, (d) glucose administration, and (e) diuretic therapy.

   Although the gastrointestinal tract can be a source of ongoing phosphorus loss, the kidney is the major organ responsible for phosphorus excretion. Phosphorus is filtered by the glomerulus and then reabsorbed mainly by the proximal tubule. This reabsorption is influenced by the factors listed above. A decrease in phosphorus intake, parathyroid hormone, and intravascular volume all increase phosphorus absorption. Independent of the effect of glucose on increasing cellular uptake, glucose directly decreases renal tubular phosphate reabsorption. Most diuretics, but especially acetazolamide, are phosphaturic.

Regulators of cellular distribution are (a) PCO_2 and pH, and (b) insulin. Respiratory alkalosis and insulin therapy result in intracellular shifts of phosphorus.
2. Conditions associated with severe acute hypophosphatemia are
   a. Chronic alcohol abuse, particularly in the setting of alcoholic ketoacidosis and caloric refeeding.
   b. Treatment of diabetic ketoacidosis.
   c. Chronic and/or heavy use of oral phosphate (PO_4) binding agents.
   d. Recovery from severe burns.
   e. Hyperalimentation without adequate PO_4 replacement.
   f. Caloric refeeding after combined calorie and phosphorus malnutrition.
   g. Severe respiratory alkalosis [1].

   The pathophysiologic mechanism responsible for the hypophosphatemia in each of the above conditions are
   a. In chronic alcoholic patients, the hypophosphatemia is multifactoral and includes (1) poor dietary intake, (2) diarrhea and malabsorption with losses of ingested phosphorus, (3) respiratory alkalosis, which is common in alcoholics with severe liver disease and in alcoholic patients in withdrawal (see below), (4) alcoholic ketoacidosis (see below), (5) refeeding with calories, which drives phosphorus into cells, presumably liver cells, in the process of glycogen synthesis (see below).
   b. Diabetic ketoacidosis is associated with hypophosphatemia because phosphorus is lost from cells and excreted in the urine during the hypoinsulemic acidosis. During therapy, phosphorus moves into cells.
   c. Binding agents make dietary phosphorus unavailable for gastrointestinal absorption.
   d. In the recovery from burns, phosphorus moves into cells, presumably during anabolism.
   e. Hyperalimentation and refeeding again represent utilization of phosphorus in cell synthesis.
   f. In severe respiratory alkalosis, but not metabolic alkalosis, phosphorus moves into cells.

   In many of these instances, hypophosphatemia is not present on admission to the hospital but occurs thereafter. In diabetic ketoacidosis, the low point usually occurs in 2 to 3 days; in alcoholics, in 2 to 4 days; in hyperalimentation, in 6 to 10 days.
3. Hypokalemia and hypomagnesemia are frequently associated with severe hypophosphatemia. In fact, hypokalemia may be a clue to hypophosphatemia in hospitalized patients, since in many institutions, the serum potassium determination is available before the results of the serum phosphorus determination.

4. The clinical consequences of severe hypophosphatemia are as follows:
   a. Red cell injury with spherocytic formation and even hemolysis—uncommon.
   b. Impaired white blood cell chemotactic, phagocytic, and bactericidal activity.
   c. Thrombocytopenia and platelet dysfunction—rarely associated with clinical bleeding diathesis.
   d. Central nervous system dysfunction ranging from irritability to coma.
   e. Rhabdomyolysis—may be the major mechanism of alcoholic rhabdomyolysis.
   f. Congestive heart failure.
   g. Metabolic acidosis—uncommon (hyperchloremic in type) [1].
5. Oral replacement is adequate if the patient's phosphorus is above 1 mg/100 ml and not associated with major sequelae. Oral replacement can be given as skim milk, 1 quart per day; Fleet enema, 15 to 30 ml 3 times a day, orally; or potassium phosphate and sodium phosphate tablets. The first two are most commonly used.

    If the patient has marked hypophosphatemia or major sequelae, intravenous replacement is desirable.

    Both sodium phosphate and potassium phosphate preparations are available. Usually, giving one-half the daily potassium replacement as potassium phosphate will prevent severe hypophosphatemia.
6. Phosphorus, like potassium, is predominately an intracellular cation. Therefore, serum values may not reflect total body stores. Hypophosphatemia can exist without phosphate depletion, and phosphate depletion can exist without hypophosphatemia. The clinical conditions associated with chronic phosphorus deficiency are
   a. Malabsorption
   b. Chronic alcohol abuse
   c. Renal tubular acidosis (proximal)
   d. Chronic use of phosphate binding antacids
   e. Vitamin D deficiency [1]
7. The clinical sequelae of chronic phosphorus deficiency are
   a. Osteomalacia with bone pain
   b. Proximal myopathy with weakness
   c. Hypercalciuria

    The osteomalacia is a direct consequence of the low serum phosphorus resulting in failure of mineralization of osteoid. The proximal myopathy may well reflect a depletion of cellular adenosine triphosphate. The mechanism of the hypercalciuria is not clear.

8. The treatment of chronic phosphate deficiency includes
   a. Elimination of the primary cause of the phosphate deficiency
   b. Increasing dietary phosphorus intake
   c. Supplemental phosphorus therapy
9. The causes of hyperphosphatemia can be divided into those that are relatively acute and those that are more chronic.
   a. Acute:
      (1) Acute renal failure
      (2) Rhabdomyolysis
      (3) Lactic acidosis
      (4) Phosphorus therapy
      (5) Chemotherapy
   b. Chronic:
      (1) Chronic renal failure
      (2) Hypoparathyroidism
      (3) Hyperthyroidism

   The mechanisms involved in some of these causes are as follows:
   a. The kidney is the major route of phosphorus excretion. Therefore, impairment of renal function (usually a glomerular filtration rate <30 ml/min) is associated with phosphorus retention.
   b. In rhabdomyolysis, muscle cells break down and/or leak their intracellular contents. Phosphate is a major intracellular anion, and therefore rhabdomyolysis frequently results in marked hyperphosphatemia, particularly if renal impairment also occurs.
   c. Lactic acidosis has been associated with hyperphosphatemia. Phosphorus levels are not as increased in ketoacidosis with comparable degrees of acidemia, suggesting that some factor other than pH is involved. However, the mechanism is not defined.
   d. Parathyroid hormone reduces distal tubular reabsorption of phosphorus, and a decrease in this hormone increases phosphorus reabsorption and hence serum levels.
   e. With the recent zeal to replace phosphorus, we have seen a number of patients develop frank hyperphosphatemia secondary to large amounts of intravenous phosphorus, usually in the setting of impaired renal function.
10. Renal failure and rhabdomyolysis are the most common causes of hyperphosphatemia. These disorders are associated with the highest serum levels, levels occasionally exceeding 10 mg/100 ml.
11. The most important factor in deciding on therapy for hyperphosphatemia is the serum calcium and the serum calcium-phosphorus product. Patients with marked hypocalcemia (serum calcium <7.0 mg/100 ml) and/or symptomatic hypocalcemia require therapy di-

rected at lowering the serum phosphorus. This would be expected to increase the serum calcium.

Statistically, a serum calcium-phosphorus product ($S_{Ca} \times S_{PO_4}$) greater than 70 is felt to be associated with increased soft tissue calcification. Therefore, the serum phosphorus concentration should be lowered in this circumstance in an attempt to minimize this complication.

12. The most common modality for treating hyperphosphatemia is an oral phosphate binding agent, such as Amphogel. Such agents bind phosphate in the gastrointestinal tract and make it unavailable for absorption. These medications plus dietary manipulation are used in management of chronic renal failure. Because of frequent concurrent problems in acute renal failure, patients may be taking nothing orally. In that setting, dialysis therapy becomes important in controlling the serum phosphorus. Also, hyperalimentation with no or limited phosphorus supplementation will result in lowering of serum phosphorus and can be utilized for that effect.

Specific Patient Problems
Patient A

A 43-year-old man with a history of chronic heavy alcohol intake was admitted to the hospital with a chief complaint of severe weakness, making it impossible for him to get out of bed. His past medical history was positive for an episode of gastrointestinal bleeding from gastritis 1 year ago. Since that time he had taken some antacid on an intermittent basis. The only abnormal physical findings that were recorded were decreased muscle tone and strength with diminished deep tendon reflexes. The patient's initial laboratory values were

Na	120 mEq/L
K	2 mEq/L
Cl	95 mEq/L
HCO$_3$	15 mEq/L

The patient was given 5% dextrose in ½ normal saline at 100 ml per hour, thiamine, and 30 mEq KCl. Twenty-four hours later, the patient developed respiratory failure requiring intubation. The patient was seen in consultation by the pulmonary service. Cardiovascular examination revealed an apical impulse that was displaced leftward and a loud left-ventricular gallop. Rales were heard bibasilarly. Chest x-ray was compatible with pulmonary edema.

1. What are the possible causes for the congestive heart failure? What are the possible causes for respiratory failure?
2. Why was it precipitated in the hospital?
3. What was the clue that this was likely to happen?
4. What is the appropriate therapy?
5. In what settings should one think of hypophosphatemia?

Patient B

R. D. is a 32-year-old man with a history of a previous suicide attempt who apparently ingested 30 Darvon tablets and was found unconscious by a friend. The ambulance was called. The patient was witnessed to have four grand mal seizures. He was intubated and given 3 ampules of Narcan in the field. An Ewald tube was inserted in the emergency room, and the patient was lavaged. Initial physical examination revealed pulse 80 per minute, respiration 24 per minute, temperature 35.9°C, blood pressure 100/70 mm Hg. Neurologic examination revealed a very lethargic man without focal signs. Initial laboratory examination revealed

Na	144 mEq/L
K	6 mEq/L
Cl	101 mEq/L
HCO_3	10 mEq/L
Blood urea nitrogen (BUN)	17 mg/100 ml
PO_4	9 mg/100 ml
Calcium (Ca)	7.4 mg/100 ml
Uric acid	11.4 mg/100 ml
Urinalysis	4+ heme; trace protein
	2–5 red blood cells per high-power field (Foley catheter in place)

1. What is the most likely cause of this patient's hyperphosphatemia?
2. What is the cause of the hyperkalemia?
3. What therapy would you direct at the hyperphosphatemia?

Solutions to Specific Patient Problems
Patient A

1. In this setting of severe chronic alcoholism, a number of possibilities for congestive heart failure need to be considered:
   a. Congestive cardiomyopathy secondary to alcohol abuse
   b. Beriberi (thiamine deficiency)
   c. Rhabdomyolysis with cardiac involvement secondary to hypokalemia, hypophosphatemia, or alcohol (rare)
   d. Congestive cardiomyopathy secondary to hypophosphatemia

   The respiratory failure with hypoxia and hypercapnia requiring intubation in this setting could be due to
   a. Pneumonia with adult respiratory distress syndrome
   b. Severe pulmonary edema secondary to primary cardiac failure
   c. Primary failure of ventilation secondary to muscle weakness resulting from hypokalemia or hypophosphatemia

   This patient was profoundly hypophosphatemic with a serum phosphorus concentration of 0.3 mg/100 ml. This undoubtedly contributed to his cardiac and respiratory failure.

2. The causative role of hypophosphatemia is suggested by the temporal sequence. Alcoholic patients are commonly phosphate-depleted, albeit with a normal serum phosphorus on admission to the hospital. Administration of calories, as 5% dextrose in water, results in the intracellular movement of phosphorus with subsequent hypophosphatemia. Usually, the time course is such that the serum phosphorus falls below 1 mg/100 ml between 2 and 4 days after admission. The cardiac symptoms and muscle weakness seem to correlate with the serum phosphorus and become manifested with a serum phosphorus less than 1 mg/100 ml.
3. The decreased serum potassium concentration is a clue to the hypophosphatemia. In the alcoholic patient, potassium and phosphorus frequently go hand in hand.
4. For severe, prolonged hypophosphatemia, the recommended dose is 0.16 mmole per kilogram parenterally over 6 hours. One may want to increase this by 20 to 50 percent because of complications of hypophosphatemia. Serum phosphorus should then be repeated and appropriate adjustments made. A potassium phosphate preparation such as K-Phos ($K_2H\ PO_4 + K\ H_2PO_4$) should be used in this patient because of simultaneous potassium depletion. In most circumstances, giving one-half the potassium replacement for the first 24 hours as K-Phos will provide an appropriate amount of phosphorus.
5. The most common setting in which to see severe hypophosphatemia is in the alcoholic patient who enters the hospital and is given caloric refeeding, is treated for ketoacidosis, and has severe respiratory alkalosis.

Patient B

1. Rhabdomyolysis is the most likely cause of the hyperphosphatemia. This may be in the presence of acute renal failure. There is not sufficient data given to make a judgment about acute renal failure at this point.

    The clinical setting of an unresponsive patient with a drug overdose is a common one for rhabdomyolysis. This probably represents ischemic muscle injury from the patient's lying in one position for a prolonged period. Recurrent seizures also are associated with rhabdomyolysis. The markedly heme-positive urine by dipstick with only 2 to 5 red blood cells per high-power field suggests myoglobin in the urine.
2. The hyperkalemia and the high uric acid also may reflect loss of cellular constituents into the serum. The patient is probably acidemic (HCO_3 10 mEq/L), and this may contribute to the hyperkalemia as well. However, it should be pointed out that the lactic acidosis secondary to seizures is not associated with hyperkalemia. Hyperuricemia, as well as hyperphosphatemia, can accompany lactic acidosis, and it is possible that this is operative to some extent in the observed increased phosphorus and uric acid. The heme-positive urine, however, makes it unlikely that lactic acidosis is the sole explanation and implicates rhabdomyolysis.

3. The initial therapy should be directed at restoring blood pressure with volume replacement and supplying adequate ventilation. Therapy should also be directed at establishing an adequate urine output. If urine output is not obtained by volume repletion alone, furosemide should be given. Establishment of a good urine output (2 L/24 hr) is the best therapy for hyperphosphatemia in this setting. If the patient is oliguric and renal failure ensues, then management as indicated for acute renal failure needs to be instituted (see Chap. 2).

Reference

Knochel, J. P. Clinical spectrum of acute and chronic phosphate depletion. Presented at the Kidney Disease and Renal Failure Symposium, Aspen, Colorado, 1978.

Suggested Reading

Alfrey, A. C. Disorders of Magnesium Metabolism. In R. W. Schrier (Ed.), *Renal and Electrolyte Disorders* (2nd ed.), Boston: Little, Brown, 1980. Pp. 299–320.

Darsee, J. R., and Nettler, D. O. Reversible severe congestive cardiomyopathy in three cases of hypophosphatemia. *Ann. Intern. Med.* 89:867, 1978.

Knochel, J. P. The pathophysiology and clinical characteristics of severe hypophosphatemia. *Arch. Intern. Med.* 137:203, 1977.

Lentz, R. D., et al. Treatment of severe hypophosphatemia. *Ann. Intern. Med.* 89:941, 1978.

10. Disorders of Magnesium Metabolism

General Questions
1. What is the distribution of magnesium in the body?
2. What factors control magnesium concentration?
3. What other cation seems to be altered by similar pathophysiologic states?
4. List the causes of hypomagnesemia, and comment on the mechanisms involved.
5. What are the clinical manifestations of hypomagnesemia?
6. What are the indications for therapy and the modalities of therapy in hypomagnesemia?
7. List the causes of hypermagnesemia.
8. What are the signs and symptoms of hypermagnesemia?
9. What are the indications for therapy in hypermagnesemia, and what modalities can be used?

Solutions to General Questions
1. Total body magnesium (Mg) is about 20 mmole per kilogram. Sixty-five percent is in bone; only a small percentage of this is rapidly exchangeable. Like potassium, most of the remaining magnesium is intracellular, with 22 percent of total magnesium in muscle cells.
2. No hormone seems to be involved in day-to-day control of magnesium. The kidney seems to be the major regulator of plasma magnesium concentration.
3. Alteration in serum potassium and serum magnesium commonly occurs together. In a clinical setting where potassium measurements may be more rapidly available, alterations in potassium should be used to suggest alterations in plasma magnesium.
4. The causes of hypomagnesemia are as follows:
   a. Redistribution
      (1) Treatment of diabetic ketoacidosis
      (2) Refeeding
      (3) Postparathyroidectomy
      In treating ketoacidosis, a similar redistribution occurs as occurs with potassium. In postparathyroidectomy, some of the redistribution may be related to bone healing.
   b. Gastrointestinal losses
      (1) Nasogastric suction (Gastric fluid is relatively high in magnesium, containing 1 mEq/L.)
      (2) Diarrhea
      (3) Malabsorption, general or specific for magnesium

c. Renal loss
   (1) Alcohol (acute)
   (2) Osmotic diuresis
   (3) Postobstructive diuresis
   (4) Hyperaldosteronism (Bartter's syndrome)
   (5) Potassium depletion
   (6) Diuretic therapy
   (7) Aminoglycoside therapy

   In the alcoholic patient, the serum magnesium correlates poorly with the degree of deficit, which may be large. The magnesium deficiency in this population is multifactoral, reflecting poor dietary intake, malabsorption, hyperaldosteronism, ketosis, increased lactate, and alcohol-induced magnesuria.

   The most magnesuric diuretics are the loop diuretics.
d. Skin loss
   (1) Burns
   (2) Sweating
5. The clinical manifestations of hypomagnesemia are as follows:
   a. Neuromuscular
      (1) Muscle fibrillation
      (2) Weakness
      (3) Ataxia
      (4) Vertigo
      (5) Nystagmus
      (6) Convulsions
      (7) Tetany
      (8) Carpal pedal spasm
   b. Cardiac
      (1) Premature ventricular contractions
      (2) Ventricular tachycardia
      (3) Ventricular fibrillation
      (4) Increased digitalis toxicity
   c. Gastrointestinal
      (1) Anorexia
      (2) Nausea
   d. Psychiatric
      (1) Apathy
      (2) Depression
      (3) Irritability
      (4) Delirium
6. Therapy should be instituted if the serum magnesium is less than 1 mEq per liter or if central nervous system, cardiac, or neuromuscular sequelae of hypomagnesemia exist.

If cardiac arrest is imminent or if severe neuromuscular dysfunction is present, 4 ml of 50% magnesium sulfate ($MgSO_4$) solution in 100 ml of saline can be given intravenously over 10 minutes. If less severe manifestations are present, 4 ml of 50% $MgSO_4$ solution can be administered intramuscularly.

7. The causes of hypermagnesemia are as follows:
   a. Increased endogenous load—catabolic states
   b. Increased intake
      (1) Magnesium-containing laxatives
      (2) Epsom salts
      (3) Excess parenteral magnesium in treating preeclampsia
   c. Decreased excretion
      (1) Renal failure
      (2) Hypothyroidism
      (3) Mineralocorticoid deficiency
8. The signs and symptoms of hypermagnesemia are as follows:

Serum Magnesium	Signs and Symptoms
> 5 mEq/L	Decreased blood pressure
> 7 mEq/L	Central nervous system depression
> 9 mEq/L	Nausea and vomiting
> 10 mEq/L	Decreased reflexes
> 10 mEq/L	Abnormal electrocardiogram, increased P–R interval, decreased QSR, decreased P wave
> 13 mEq/L	Decreased respirations
> 13 mEq/L	Coma
> 16 mEq/L	Cardiac arrest

If shock occurs from hypermagnesemia, the patient should have no deep tendon reflexes. If reflexes are present, another cause should be considered.

9. If no symptoms are present with serum magnesium 5 mEq per liter or less, intake should be decreased and the underlying cause attacked.

If respiratory depression, cardiac conduction defect, or hypotension exists, more decisive measures are needed. In these cases, 2.5 to 5.0 mmole of calcium intravenously and insulin and glucose, which will drive magnesium into cells (same as potassium), should be given. Saline infusion and loop diuretics could be tried, although sparse data on their efficacy are available. Dialysis will effectively remove excess magnesium.

Specific Patient Problems
Patient A

An 87-year-old man was admitted for evaluation of constipation, anemia, and a positive Hemoccult test of stools of 1-month duration. Past history was significant for myocardial infarction, chronic atrial fibrillation with slow ventricular response, congestive heart failure, and intermittent claudication. His medications were furosemide, potassium chloride, isosorbide dinitrate, hydralazine, and ferrous sulfate.

Physical examination showed an elderly cachectic man in no distress. The blood pressure was 130/70 mm Hg, pulse rate 62 per minute, and respirations 22 per minute. Physical findings included an elevated jugular venous pressure, scattered bibasilar rales, cardiomegaly, and a Grade II/VI mitral regurgitant murmur. The liver span was 12 cm. There were multiple soft masses throughout the abdomen consistent with stool in the colon. The rectum disclosed no masses but was packed with firm stool.

On admission the hematocrit was 35% and white blood cell count 8,700. The blood urea nitrogen was 30 mg/100 ml, creatinine 1.6 mg/100 ml, and calcium 10 mg/100 ml. Serum electrolytes and albumin were normal.

A barium enema was scheduled, and soap suds enemas were administered. The patient was to receive an oral dose of 300 ml of magnesium citrate. However, when magnesium citrate was unavailable, 300 ml of the standard solution of magnesium sulfate was substituted.

Shortly thereafter the patient developed nausea and vomiting. Within a few hours, copious watery diarrhea was noted. The patient complained of chest pain and was found to be hypotensive and bradycardic. The electrocardiogram is shown below.

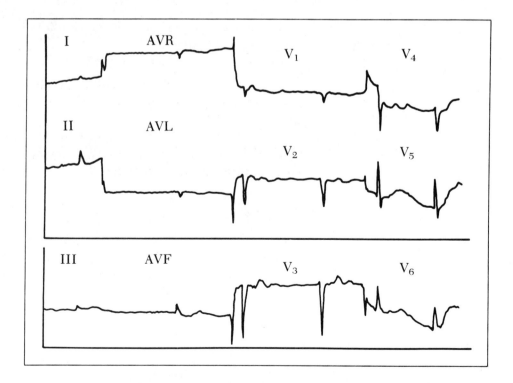

Initially, heart rate and hypotension showed some improvement with atropine and intravenous fluids. However, refractory hypotension and bradycardia returned. The cardiology service was consulted and felt the patient had a myocardial infarction. The patient expired several hours later.

1. What was the magnesium load that the patient received?
2. What events were responsible for the bradycardia and hypotension?
3. How could the diagnosis of magnesium intoxication be made at the bedside?
4. What is the immediate and definitive therapy?

Patient B

C. T. was a 38-year-old woman admitted for abdominal pain, after being hit with a lead pipe, and increasing jaundice. Her pertinent history included heavy alcohol intake for 19 years with four admissions for withdrawal, one for alcoholic ketoacidosis, and one for cirrhosis.

The patient developed fever with bilateral pulmonary infiltrates and persistent diarrhea. Six weeks later, the patient's sputum cultures confirmed a diagnosis of tuberculosis, and treatment was started with streptomycin, ethambutol, and rifampin.

One week later, the patient developed carpopedal spasm. Both Chvostek's and Trousseau's signs could be demonstrated.

The patient's laboratory data at that time were

Na	136 mEq/L	Creatinine	0.4 mg/100 ml
K	3 mEq/L	Calcium (Ca)	4.5 mg/100 ml
Cl	100 mEq/L	Phosphate (PO_4)	4.6 mg/100 ml
HCO_3	22 mEq/L	Total protein	6.7 gm/100 ml
BUN	3 mEq/L	Albumin	2 gm/100 ml

The patient was treated with intravenous fluids, including calcium gluconate and potassium. Magnesium was also given for several days and then discontinued.

Five days later the patient was found agonal; intubation was complicated by marked laryngospasm. Cardiac arrest occurred, and the patient could not be resuscitated.

1. What is the most likely cause of the carpopedal spasm and positive Chvostek's and Trousseau's signs?
2. Can the hypocalcemia be explained by the hypoalbuminemia?
3. What laboratory test would you order at this point?
4. Why do you think this patient was hypomagnesemic?

5. How would you treat this patient? As stated, the patient was given calcium gluconate intravenously. Would you agree with that therapy? Why?
6. What do you think was responsible for the patient's terminal event?
7. What therapy would you have given during the attempted resuscitation?

Solutions to Specific Patient Problems
Patient A

1. The standard dose of magnesium citrate for laxation in adults is 300 ml. This is a 16% solution and contains 3.2 gm of elemental magnesium. This patient received 300 ml of 61% solution of magnesium sulfate, containing 17.8 gm of elemental magnesium.
2. Magnesium salts are classified as saline cathartics. The laxative mechanism appears to be the intraluminal accumulation of water and electrolytes due to an osmotic effect of the poorly absorbable magnesium ion. The initial hypotension undoubtedly reflected the osmotic movement of fluid from the extracellular fluid to the gut. With the osmotic load delivered, 2 to 3 liters of fluid would be withdrawn from the extracellular fluid. Magnesium citrate, the usual magnesium cathartic, is not hypertonic as was the solution the patient received, and therefore this massive fluid shift usually does not occur.

    Oral or parenteral loads of magnesium normally are rapidly excreted by the kidneys. Magnesium excretion is enhanced in states of volume expansion and reduced in most azotemic states. This patient's mild azotemia and probable volume depletion secondary to vomiting and excessive osmotic diarrhea likely compromised his ability to excrete the magnesium load.

    The serum magnesium increased, and magnesium intoxication occurred. Physiologic consequences of hypermagnesemia ensued from the pharmacologic effects of the magnesium ion on the nervous and cardiovascular systems (see General Problems, above).

    Magnesium cardiotoxicity was the most likely cause of the death in this patient. It should also be noted that, in the setting of renal insufficiency, clinical cardiotoxicity may be seen with only modest elevations of serum magnesium.
3. Loss of deep tendon reflexes occurs at 10 mEq per liter. If deep tendon reflexes had been present initially and then lost, magnesium intoxication should have been diagnosed.

4. The therapy for hypermagnesium in this setting includes
   a. Intravenous calcium as the immediate treatment. Calcium gluconate (15 mg of calcium/kg) can be administered over 4-hour periods to produce a calciuresis and thus hypermagnesuria.
   b. If renal function is adequate, intravenous furosemide with saline replacement of urinary losses should be instituted. If renal function is not adequate, hemodialysis should be instituted.

Patient B

1. The hypocalcemia is responsible for these findings.
2. The fact that the patient is exhibiting clinical evidence of hypocalcemia means that the decrease in calcium reflects not only a decrease in protein-bound calcium, as occurs in hypoalbuminemia, but also a decrease in ionized, or physiologically active, calcium as well. In addition, using the rough rule of thumb, raising the albumin by 2 to 4 gm/100 ml would only raise the calcium from 4.5 to 6.5 (4.5 + 2.0) mg/100 ml, which is still clearly low (see Chap. 8 and 9).
3. A serum magnesium level test should be ordered at this point. The result was 0.5 mEq per liter.
4. The patient had multiple reasons for hypomagnesemia and magnesium depletion.
   a. Chronic alcoholism with its accompanying poor dietary intake, intermittently increased urinary excretion during withdrawal, and frequently, malabsorption.
   b. Diarrhea with gastrointestinal losses.
   c. Prolonged intravenous therapy without magnesium replacement.
   d. Renal losses secondary to aminoglycoside therapy.
5. As the patient was having marked carpopedal spasm with a very low calcium, parenteral therapy with magnesium is indicated.

    One gram of $MgSO_4$ = 8 mEq Mg = 4 mmole Mg = 2 ml 50% $MgSO_4$.

    Four milliliters of 50% $MgSO_4$ or 16 mEq could be given in 100 ml of fluid over half an hour, and 3 ml of 50% $MgSO_4$ intravenously, daily for 3 days.

    If the patient were not a debilitated alcoholic with a prolonged prothrombin time, the magnesium could be given intramuscularly as 2 ml of 50% $MgSO_4$ in each buttock every 4 hours for 24 hours, followed by 2 ml intramuscularly 4 times a day for 3 days.

    Calcium administration will not significantly improve hypocalcemia in a hypomagnesemic patient.

6. The patient most likely developed recurrent hypomagnesemia and subsequent hypocalcemia. The laryngospasm suggests this.
7. Magnesium was not given during the resuscitation but should have been. In this setting of cardiac arrest, 10 ml of 20% $MgSO_4$ can be given intravenously over 1 minute (see General Questions, above).

Suggested Reading

Alfrey, A. C. Disorders of Magnesium Metabolism. In R. W. Schrier (Ed.), *Renal and Electrolyte Disorders* (2nd ed.). Boston: Little, Brown, 1980. Pp. 299–320.

Shils, M. E. Experimental human magnesium depletion. *Medicine* 48:61, 1969.

Index

Abuse
  alcohol. *See also* Ketoacidosis, alcoholic
    anion gap metabolic acidosis, 25, 36, 51, 86
    congestive heart failure, 112
    hypomagnesemia, 116, 121
    hypophosphatemia, 108, 113
    pancreatitis, 36
  solvent abuse, metabolic complications of, 88–89

Acetest
  interpretation of, 1, 4, 5
  use of in detecting ketosis, 24, 25, 36, 51

Acid-base, approach to analysis of disorder, 31

Acidification, mechanism of for urine, 2, 27–28

Acidosis
  anion gap, 30–31, 35–42
    alcoholic, causes in alcoholic patient, 36. *See also* Ketoacidosis
    alkalemia, meaning of anion gap in, 50–51
    causes of, 24, 25, 35, 36, 85, 86, 105
    diabetic. *See* Diabetic ketoacidosis
    ethylene glycol intoxication, 25, 51, 86
    lactic. *See* Lactic acidosis
    methanol intoxication, 25, 51, 86
    renal failure, 15, 25, 105
    salicylate intoxication, 51, 86

Acidosis, cerebral spinal fluid pH in, 34, 35

Acidosis, hyperchloremic, 29–35
  aldosterone, deficiency in, 26, 32
  carbonic anhydrase inhibition in, 26, 32
  causes, 26, 32, 33, 64, 88, 94, 95
  diarrhea, 26, 32, 88
  phosphorus deficiency as cause, 109
  PTH, 95
  renal tubular acidosis, 26, 28, 29, 32, 33, 88
  urinary pH, use in, 2, 3, 32, 33, 88

Acidosis, metabolic
  definition of, 23
  carbon dioxide in, 27

Acidosis, potassium, effect of, 33, 36, 80, 85

Acidosis, respiratory
  hypermagnesemia, as cause of, 117
  hypokalemia, as cause of, 39, 112
  hypophosphatemia, as cause of, 112

Acidosis, respiratory compensation for, 32, 35, 49, 86

Acidosis, treatment of
  anion gap type, 38
  bicarbonate therapy for, 34, 37, 38, 87, 89
  CSF acidosis during, 34–35
  hyperchloremic, 34
  lactic acidosis from, 37

Acute renal failure (ARF), 9–22
  anemia in, 16
  causes, 10, 20, 50, 73, 86, 87
  complications, 16–17, 22, 25, 80, 99, 110, 117
  contraindicated drugs in, 18
  definition, 9
  dialysis for, 18
  differential diagnosis for, 9, 10–15 (table)
  furosemide therapy in, indications for, 21
  historical data in, 10–13 (table)
  laboratory data in, 10–13 (table), 15 (table)
  management, 17–18
  mannitol, use of, 21
  non-oliguric, 16
  oliguria, 19
  physical examination in, 10–13
  radiographic techniques in diagnosis, 16
  signs of, 10–13 (table)
  symptoms in, 10–13 (table)
  urinalysis in, 14 (table)
  urine chemistries in diagnosing, 18, 22, 73

Addison's disease, 81. *See also* Adrenal insufficiency

Adenosine monophosphate (AMP), cyclic, 93
  in tests for hypercalcemia, 96

ADH. *See* Antidiuretic hormone

Adrenal insufficiency, 59, 63, 64, 94

AKA. *See* Ketoacidosis, alcoholic

Albumin
  effect on anion gap in alkalemia, 50

Albumin—*Continued*
  effect on serum calcium, 92, 97–98, 99 (figure), 104, 121
  urine dipstick test for, 3
Aldosterone
  in potassium metabolism, 81
  role in metabolic alkalosis, 45–47
Alkalemia
  effect on calcium, 105
  severe, treatment for, 52–53
Alkalosis, metabolic, 43–55
  acetazolamide as treatment for, 53
  arginine monohydrochloride as treatment for, 53
  causes, 44–45, 50
  classification of, 44
  definitions, 43
  diuretic induced, 46–47
  gastric outlet obstruction induced, 55
  generation of, 43, 45–47
  hydrochloric acid in treatment of, 52
  hyperaldosteronism. *See* Mineralocorticoid
  hypoventilation in treatment of, 52
  increased anion gap in, 26, 53
  lysine monohydrochloride in treatment of, 53
  milk-alkali syndrome, 45, 50
  mineralocorticoid excess, induced, 47–48
  phosphorus in, 105
  pre-renal azotemia, 15, 50, 54
  respiratory compensation for, 46, 49, 52, 54
  sodium-chloride responsive, 44–45
  sodium-chloride unresponsive, 45
  treatment, 52–53
  vomiting induced, 44–46
  urinary chloride in classification, 44
Alkalosis, respiratory
  alcoholism and, 108, 113
  causes of, 51
  hypokalemia in, 77, 78
  hypophosphatemia in, 108
Amino aciduria
  RTA and, 29
  urinary dipstick for protein and, 29
AMP. *See* Adenosine monophosphate
Amyloidosis, 16
Anion gap. *See* Acidosis; Alkalosis

Anorexia, hypercalcemia and, 96
Antidiuretic hormone (ADH)
  central diabetes insipidus and, 70
  glucocorticoid deficiency and, 59
  hyponatremia and, 51–61, 63–66
  nephrogenic DI and, 70
  syndrome of inappropriate secretion of (SIADH), 59–61, 63–66, 85
  volume stimulated release of, 59, 84
ARF. *See* Acute renal failure
Arrhythmias, cardiac
  alkalemia and, 49, 53
  hyperkalemia and, 81, 83, 87
  hypermagnesemia, 117, 120
  hypocalcemia, 100
  hypokalemia and, 80
  hypomagnesemia, 116, 122
Azotemia, prerenal (PRA)
  differential diagnosis, 9–15, 20–21, 33, 50, 73, 104
  laboratory data in, 10–13
  signs and symptoms of, 10–13
  urinalysis in, 15
  urinary chemistries in, 16

Bence Jones protein, 3
Bicarbonate
  correcting excess, 52
  in diabetic ketoacidosis, 37, 38
  in diagnosis
    of acid-base disturbances, 31
    of ARF, 15 (table)
    of metabolic acidosis, 23
  disorders of potassium metabolism and, 82 (table), 85
  hyperbicarbonatemia in renal disorders, 10, 11 (table)
  hyperchloremic acidosis and, 24, 34
  metabolic acidosis and, 46, 49
    alkalemia, 35
    cerebrospinal fluid acidosis, 34
    therapy for, 33, 34, 35, 38
  proximal or distal RTA and, 28, 29, 32, 33
  PTH and, 95
  resorption of, 27–28, 44 (table)
  respiratory alkalosis and, 49
  serum, concentration
    in alcoholic ketoacidosis, 4
    in anion gap acidosis, 53
    in gastric outlet obstruction, 55
    in metabolic alkalosis, 43–44, 50
    in tumor-related hypercalcemia, 95
  vomiting and, 47

in SIADH, 64
urine pH and, 2
Blood urea nitrogen (BUN)
ARF and, 22, 85
BUN/creatinine ratio, 13
contraindicated drugs and, 18
CRF and, 32
in diagnosis, 10–11 (table), 13, 25 (table), 33, 87
of ARF, 9
of hypernatremia, 73
of hyperosmolar states, 73
of hypocalcemia, 99 (table), 104
of PRA, 21, 33, 104
of SIADH, 64
dialysis and, 18
as indicator of GFR, 21
protein intake and, 13, 88
Bone
osteomalacia, 109
vitamin D absorption and, 92–93
BUN. *See* Blood urea nitrogen

Calcitonin
and calcium homeostasis, 92
and hypocalcemia, 98
Calcium
homeostasis, 92
hypercalcemia
differential diagnosis, 93–94
difference from hyperparathyroidism, 94 (table)
laboratory tests for, 95–96
physical examination findings for, 95
systems affected by, 96
therapy for, 97, 103
hypermagnesium, treatment for, 121
hypocalcemia
causes, 98
differential diagnosis of, 104
evaluation of, 99
signs and symptoms of, 99
therapy for, 100, 104, 110–111
hypokalemia and, 88
serum, composition of, 92
as treatment for hyperkalemia, 41 (table), 82 (table)
Calyceal system evaluation, 16
Cardiac function
in alkalemia, 53
cardiac arrest, and magnesium therapy, 122
cardiac conduction defect, in hypermagnesemia therapy, 117
cardiovascular sequelae in hypokalemia, 79, 80
congestive heart failure
and emergency dialysis, in ARF, 18
in hyponatremia, 59
in hypophosphatemia, 109, 112, 113
in PRA, 33
and total body potassium deficits, 78
in hypercalcemia, 96
in hypocalcemia, 100
in hypomagnesemia, 116, 117
magnesium cardiotoxicity, 120
in PRA, 10, 11 (table)
Cast(s), urinary, 6
broad, 6
granular, 6
hyaline, 6
RBC, 6
RTC, 6
waxy, 6
WBC, 6
Cells, in urinary sediment
epithelial, 5
red blood, 6
renal tubular epithelial, 5
white blood, 5
Central nervous system (CNS)
in causes of SIADH, 61, 85
in hypercalcemia, 97
in hypermagnesemia, 117
in hypocalcemia, 104
hyponatremia and, 63, 66
in hypophosphatemia, 109
indications for dialysis in ARF and, 18
in respiratory alkalosis, 51
substance intoxication and, 86
Cerebrospinal fluid (CSF)
acidosis, 34
bicarbonate and, 37, 55
pH of, 35
Chloride
compounds, as therapy for metabolic alkalosis, 52
in hyperchloremic acidosis, 24, 26 (table), 32
loss in vomitus, 45
serum, in hyperkalemia, 86
urine, concentration, 44
Cholecalciferol (vitamin D_3), 93
Chronic renal failure (CRF), 9
Concentration of urine. *See* Urine
CPK. *See* Creatinine, phosphokinase
Creatinine
ARF and, 9, 21, 22
cause of elevated BUN and, 88
clearance, 13

Creatinine—*Continued*
  phosphokinase (CPK), 21, 88
  serum, in PRA, 54
CRF. *See* Chronic renal failure
Crystals
  calcium oxalate, 7
  cystine, 7
  hippuric acid, 7
  uric acid, 7
CSF. *See* Cerebrospinal fluid

Dehydration, in hyperosmolar states, 70
Demeclocycline, and SIADH, 65
Diabetes
  ECG, and hypokalemia, 40
  hyporeninemic hypoaldosteronism and, 81
  insipidus
    central, 70, 71, 73
    congenital, 71
    nephrogenic, 70–71, 73
    partial, 73
  mellitus, 11 (table)
  metabolic acidosis and
    diabetic ketoacidosis, 50. *See also* Diabetic ketoacidosis (DKA)
    differential diagnosis, 36
  potassium deficits and, 78
Diabetic ketoacidosis (DKA)
  bicarbonate therapy, for potassium deficit, 37, 38
  caused by infection, 39
  hypomagnesemia and, 115
  hypophosphatemia and, 108
  saline deficit and, 37
Dialysis
  ARF and, 18, 22
  hypercalcemia and, 97 (table)
  hyperkalemia and, 42, 82
  hypermagnesemia and, 117, 121
  hyperphosphatemia, 111
Diarrhea
  hypercalcemia and, 94
  hyperchloremic acidosis and, 26 (table), 32
  hypomagnesemia and, 120
  hypokalemia and, 77, 79 (figure), 88
  hypomagnesemia and, 115, 121
  sodium loss with, 59 (table), 70 (table)
Diet
  in ARF, 17, 20, 22
  hypophosphatemia and, 108, 113
  low BUN and, 88
Digitalis, hypocalcemia therapy and, 100

2,3-Diphosphoglycerate, 37
"Dipstick proteinuria," 3
Dipstick test. *See* Urine
Diuretics
  hypokalemia and, 78
  hyponatremia and, 59 (table), 61, 66
  magnesium-wasting, 116
  metabolic alkalosis, 45, 46–47
  potassium-sparing, 81
  thiazide
    hypercalcemia and, 93
    hyponatremia and, 59
DKA. *See* Diabetic ketoacidosis
Drug-induced conditions
  ARF, 18
  hypercalcemia, 93
  hyperkalemia, 80
  hyperphosphatemia, 110
  hypokalemia, 78
  nephrogenic diabetes insipidus, 71
Dysfunction, renal
  causes, 10–13 (with table)
  serum chemistry and, 15 (table)
  urinalysis and, 14 (table)

ECF. *See* Extracellular fluid
ECG. *See* Electrocardiogram
Edema
  cerebral, replacing water loss and, 74–75
  pulmonary, 39, 54, 61
Electrocardiogram (ECG)
  in hypercalcemia, 96
  in hyperkalemia, 41, 80, 81, 82
  in hypermagnesemia, 117
  in hypocalcemia, 100
  in hypokalemia, 40, 79, 80, 89
  in hypomagnesemia, 116
Endocrine disorders, and hypercalcemia, 94
Erythematosus, systemic lupus, and potassium secretion, 81
Ethacrynic acid, and Henle's loop, 59
Ethylene glycol, and metabolic acidosis, 25 (table), 36, 86
Extracellular fluid (ECF)
  depletion of, 47, 120
  in hyperglycemia, 57
  in metabolic acidosis, 33, 36
  in metabolic alkalosis, 44 (table)

Furosemide, 21
  and Henle's loop, 59
  hypermagnesium and, 121
  hyponatremia and, 61, 66–67

Gastric drainage, and metabolic alkalosis, 55
Gastrointestinal losses
 of bicarbonate, in metabolic acidosis, 26 (table)
 of potassium, 77, 78, 79
Glomerular disease, and chronic renal failure, 10
Glomerular filtration rate (GFR)
 in ARF, 17
 in hyperphosphatemia, 110
 in hyponatremia, 17, 58, 59
 and potassium, in chronic renal failure, 81
Glomerulonephritis
 acute, 6, 13
 and ARF, 10
 chronic, 14 (table), 104
Glucocorticoid deficiency, in hyponatremia, 59
Glucose
 dipstick test, 5
 serum
  in hyponatremia, 63, 65–66
  in DKA, 36
Glucosuria, 5
Glycosuria, proximal RTA and, 29

Hematest, stool, 22
Hematuria, 2 (table), 6
Hemodialysis
 in hypermagnesemia, 121
 prophylactic, in ARF, 22
Hemoglobinuria, 3
Hemolysis, and potassium, 81
HHNK. See Hyperglycemic hyperosmolar nonketotic coma
Hormone, parathyroid (PTH). See Parathyroid hormone
Hormone, thyroid-stimulating (TSH), 103
Hormone, thyrotropin-releasing (TRH), 103
Hydrochlorothiazide, hypercalcemia and, 103
Hyperaldosteronism, 81
Hyperalimentation
 acute hypophosphatemia and, 108
 in hyperphosphatemia therapy, 111
Hypercalcemia
 causes, 93–94
 emergency states, 97
 laboratory tests for causes, 95–96
 physical examination for causes, 95
 signs and symptoms, 96
 therapy, 97 (table), 103
 tumor-related, hyperparathyroidism and, 94 (table), 98
Hypercalciuria, 29
Hypercapnia
 hypophosphatemia and, 112
 metabolic alkalosis and, 44
Hyperglycemia, 5
 glucose in, 57
Hyperglycemic hyperosmolar nonketotic coma (HHNK), 85
 glucose in, 87
 therapy aims, 69
Hyperkalemia, 105
 cardiac effects, 41, 81, 83
 causes, 80–81
 hyponatremia and, 64
 sequelae, 81
 therapy, 82 (table), 87
 uremia and, 78
 uric acid and, 113
Hyperlipidemia, 58
 pseudohyponatremia and, 57, 58
Hypermagnesemia
 cardiotoxicity and, 120
 causes, 117
 signs and symptoms, 117
 therapy, 117, 121
Hypernatremia
 categories, 70 (table)
 $NaHCO_3$ and, 34
Hyperosmolarity, HHNK therapy and, 69
Hyperparathyroidism
 hypercalcemia and, 93, 95
 PTH and, 95, 96
 tumor-related hypercalcemia, 94 (table)
Hyperphosphatemia, 105
 acute, causes, 110
 chronic, causes, 110
 hypocalcemia treatment and, 100
 mechanisms of causes, 110
 therapy, 114
Hyperproteinemia, pseudohyponatremia and, 57, 58
Hypertension, in hypercalcemia, 95
Hyperthyroidism, hypercalcemia and, 95, 103
Hypertonicity, $NaHCO_3$ and, 34
Hypertrophy, prostatic, 20
 elevated creatinine and, 50
 OU and, 20
Hyperuricemia, lactic acidosis in chronic alcoholics and, 113
Hyperuricosuria, 7
Hypoalbuminemia
 hypocalcemia and, 98
 proteinuria and, 104

Hypoaldosteronism, hyporeninemic, 28, 32
Hypocalcemia
  acute, treatment, 100
  causes, 98
  chronic, treatment, 100
  evaluation, 99
  signs and symptoms, 99–100
Hypokalemia
  cardiac effects, 79
  causes, 77–78
  complications, 80
  ECG in, 40
  hypophosphatemia and, 108
  metabolic alkalosis and, 54
  sequelae, 79–80
  treatment, 80
  urine potassium as diagnostic aid, 79
Hypomagnesemia
  causes, 115–116, 121
  clinical manifestations, 116
  hypocalcemia and, 98
  hypokalemia and, 88
  hypophosphatemia and, 108
  therapy, 116–117
Hyponatremia
  categories, 59–60 (table)
  mechanisms, 63–65, 84–85
  pathogenesis, 64
Hypophosphatemia, 93
  acute, conditions associated with, 108
  alcoholism and, 113
  clinical consequences, 109
  diabetic ketoacidosis and, 39
  hypokalemia and, 88, 108
  hypomagnesemia and, 108
  metabolic alkalosis and, 54
  osteomalacia and, 109
  pathophysiologic mechanisms responsible for, 108
  potassium phosphate as therapy, 89
  proximal RTA and, 29
Hypotension
  hypermagnesemia and, 120
  insulin and, 37
  orthostatic
    in hypercalcemia, 95
    in hypernatremia, 73
    water loss and, 74
Hypouricemia, proximal RTA and, 29
Hypoventilation, in metabolic alkalosis, 54. See also Respiratory acidosis

ICF. See Intracellular fluid
Immobilization, hypercalcemia and, 94
Insulin
  in diabetic ketoacidosis, 37, 38
  effect on glucose, 70
  in hypokalemia, 79
  phosphorus and, 108
  as regulator of serum potassium, 80
  in treatment of hyperkalemia, 82 (table), 87
Intoxication. See also specific substances
  digitalis, serum potassium and, 81
  magnesium, 120
Intracellular fluid (ICF), hyponatremia and, 57

Kayexalate, in hyperkalemia, 42, 82, 87
Keratopathy, band, in hyperparathyroidism, 95
Ketoacidosis, 24
  alcoholic (AKA), 4, 36
    serum bicarbonate and, 85
  diabetic (DKA), 4, 36
    hypophosphatemia and, 108
    metabolic acidosis and, 50
    potassium and, 37
    serum bicarbonate and, 85
    therapy aims, 69
    treatment, 37–38, 39
  hypophosphatemia in alcoholism and, 113
Ketoacids, 4
Ketones
  serum, in diagnosing anion gap acidosis, 88
  urinary, 4
Ketonomia, paraldehyde and, 86
Ketosticks, 4
Kidney. See also Dialysis; Renal failure
  Acetazolamide and, 53
  bicarbonate generation and, 28
  disease, polycystic, 16
  diuretics and NaCl reabsorption and, 46
  glucose reabsorption capacity and, 5
  in hypercalcemia, 96
  in hypokalemia, 78, 80
  in hyponatremia, 58–59
  limitation of excretions, in oliguric renal failure, 22
  magnesium regulation and, 115, 120, 121
  myeloma kidney, and acid urine, 3
  phosphorus excretion and, 107, 110

in proximal and distal RTA, 28, 29
PTH and, 93
renal calculi, 94 (table)
renal HCO_3 wasting, in hyperchloremic acidosis, 26 (table)
renal tubular epithelial cells (RTCs), 5
in SIADH, 60, 65
size, in diagnosis, 16
urinary casts and, 6

Lactic acidosis, 4, 5, 24 (table)
acute hyperphosphatemia and, 110
as cause of metabolic acidosis, 51
from seizures, 85
terminal, in DKA, 51
Lactic dehydrogenase (LDH), 21
diagnosis of myoglobinemia and, 88
Lipids, and hyponatremia, 58
Lithium, and nephrogenic DI, 71

Macroglobulinemias, 58
Magnesium
distribution, 115
hypermagnesemia
causes, 117
consequences, 120
signs and symptoms, 117
treatment, 117, 120
hypokalemia and, 88
hypomagnesemia
in alcoholics, 116, 121
calcium absorption in, 121–122
causes, 115–116
consequences, 116
treatment, 116–117, 121, 122
Malabsorption
in chronic phosphorus deficiency, 109
in hypocalcemia, 98, 99 (table)
in hypomagnesemia, 115, 116, 121
in hypophosphatemia, 108
Mannitol, 21, 87
Methanol, metabolic acidosis from, 25 (table), 36, 51, 86
Milk-alkali syndrome
and alkalosis, 45
and CRF, 50
and hypercalcemia, 94
Mineralocorticoid, hormone
in hypermagnesemia, 117
in hypokalemia, 78
in metabolic alkalosis, 45, 47
Morphine, 53, 61
Myoglobinemia, 88
Myoglobinuria, 3

NADH/NAD ratio, 4
Neoplasms, hypercalcemia and, 93
Nephrocalcinosis, and distal RTA, 29
Nephrolithiasis, and distal RTA, 29
Nephropathy
diabetic, 16
sarcoid, 16
urate, 16
Neuromuscular disorders
in hyperkalemia, 81, 82
in hypokalemia, 79
in hypophosphatemia, 113
in magnesium depletion, 116, 117
Normokalemia, potassium deficit and, 78

Obstructive uropathy (OU)
diagnosis, 20
PRA and, 9, 13
radiographic evidence for, 16
renal dysfunction and, 10, 11–12 (table)
serum chemistries, 15 (table)
urinalysis and, 14 (table)
Oliguria, 9, 16
Osmolality
serum
in hyperkalemia, 88
in hyperosmolar states, 69 (table)
in hyponatremia, 57–58, 61
urine
in ARF, 16, 22
in differential diagnosis, 50
in hyperosmolar states, 73
in hyponatremia, 60, 65
and specific gravity, 2
Osmolar gap
in metabolic acidosis, 25 (table), 36
in metabolic alkalosis, 51
Osmotic diuresis
HHNK and, 69
hypernatremia and, 70 (table)
hypokalemia and, 78, 79 (table)
PRA and, 87
Osteomalacia, in chronic phosphorus deficiency, 109
Oxalate crystals, and ethylene glycol intoxication, 7, 25 (table), 51

Pancreatitis, acute
alcoholism and, 36, 51
hypocalcemia and, 98
Papilledema, and hypervitaminosis A, 95

Paraldehyde
　ketonomia and, 86
　metabolic acidosis and, 25 (table)
Paralysis
　in hyperkalemia, 80, 81
　in hypokalemia, 78, 79, 80
　respiratory muscle, potassium and, 35, 40
Parathyroid gland, 98
　hyperparathyroidism
　　hypercalcemia and, 93, 94, 95, 96
　　hyperchloremic acidosis and, 26 (table)
　　radiographic evidence and, 95
　hypoparathyroidism, 98, 99
　pseudohypoparathyroidism, 98, 99
Parathyroid hormone (PTH)
　bicarbonate resorption and, 95
　calcium homeostasis and, 92–93
　deficiency, as cause of hypoparathyroidism, 98
　effects on serum calcium, 93
　hypercalcemia and, 93, 103
　hyperchloremic acidosis and, 26 (table), 95
　hypomagnesemia and, 98
　phosphaturia and, 93
　phosphorus absorption and, 107, 110
　serum, and hyperparathyroidism, 96
　in tests for hypercalcemia, 95, 96
pH
　in acid-base disturbance, 31
　in alkalemia, 49
　alteration, 52
　CSF, 35, 37
　defense of
　　in metabolic acidosis, 36
　　in metabolic alkalosis, 52, 53
　methods of lowering, 53
　potassium and, 78
　　hyperkalemia, 85
　　hypokalemia, 78, 79, 88
　serum, in hypokalemia, 79
　urine, in RTA, 88
Pheochromocytoma, in hypercalcemia, 95
Phosphate deficiency, hypercalcemia and, 94
Phosphate therapy, in hypophosphatemia, 109, 110, 113
Phosphaturia, PTH and, 93
Phosphorus
　bone disease and, 109
　chronic alcoholism and, 113
　dietary, 108
　oral replacement, 109
　serum
　　concentration, 109
　　diabetic ketoacidosis and, 38
　　hyperphosphatemia therapy and, 111–112
　　hypocalcemia and, 104
　　hypokalemia, 88
　　hypophosphatemia therapy and, 110
　　regulators, 107–108
　　rhabdomyolysis and, 88
Phosphorus deficiency, chronic
　clinical consequences, 109
　treatment, 110
Polyuria
　in DI, 71
　in hypercalcemia, 96
　in hypokalemia, 80
　in OU, 13
Posttransplantation, potassium deficiency and, 80, 81
Potassium. See also Hyperkalemia; Hypokalemia
　aldosterone and, 79, 80, 81
　chronic alcoholism and, 113
　in DKA, 38
　diuretics and, 78
　gastrointestinal losses of, 77, 78, 79
　in hyperchloremic metabolic acidosis treatment, 89
　magnesium and, 115
　respiratory acidosis and, 40
　urine
　　loss in, 79
　　as diagnostic aid, 79
　　urine pH in RTA and, 88
Potassium, serum, 32
　acidemia and, 33
　hypophosphatemia and, 108
　metabolic acidosis and, 35, 36
　metabolic alkalosis and, 46
　in pseudohyperkalemia, 81
　regulators, 80
Protein
　serum, 6
　　alkalemia and, 50
　urinary, 3, 6
Proteinuria, 3, 6, 11 (table), 14 (table)
　hypoalbuminemia, 14
Pseudohyperkalemia, 80
Pseudohypocalcemia, 98
Pseudohyponatremia
　causes, 57
　macroglobulinemias and, 58
　serum glucose in, 63
Pseudohypoparathyroidism, 98, 99

Pseudoketosis, paraldehyde and, 86
Pyuria, 6

Radiography
  in hypercalcemia, 95
  in milk-alkali syndrome, 50
  in renal failure, 16
Renal failure. *See also* Kidney; Obstructive uropathy (OU)
  acute (ARF). *See also* Acute renal failure
    causes, 10, 10–13 (table)
    hyperphosphatemia and, 114
    postrenal azotemia and, 9, 15
    prerenal azotemia and, 9, 10, 13, 15, 20
    protein and calorie intake and, 17, 20
    urinalysis and, 5, 6, 14 (table), 16
  anion gap and, 85
  chronic (CRF)
    causes, 10, 10–13 (table)
    calcium and 15 (table)
    nephrogenic DI and, 70
  differential diagnosis of, 14 (table), 15 (table), 33, 50, 51, 73, 104
  hypercalcemia and, 94, 96
  hyperkalemia and, 80, 81, 105
  hypermagnesemia and, 117
  in hyperosmolar states, 73
  hyperphosphatemia and, 110, 111, 114
  hypokalemia and, 80
  metabolic acidosis and, 25 (table), 32
  metabolic alkalosis and, 51, 54
  radiography in, 16
  serum bicarbonate and, 85
  serum creatinine level and, 50
Renal failure index (RFI), 22
Renal tubular acidosis (RTA). *See also* Renal failure
  distal, 28, 29, 32
  proximal, 28, 29, 32, 33
  urine pH in, 88
"Reset osmostat," 64
Respiratory disturbances
  differential diagnosis, 32, 54
  respiratory acidosis
    and hypocalcemia, 40
    and normal PCO_2, 39
    respiratory compensation, in acidemia, 40
  respiratory alkalosis
    causes of, 51, 54
    and hypokalemia, 78
    and hypophosphatemia, 108, 112, 113
    and metabolic acidosis, 25 (table), 35
    and metabolic alkalosis, 49
    respiratory muscle weakness, and decreased potassium, 34
RFI. *See* Renal failure index
Rhabdomyolysis, 21, 22
  ARF and, 20, 21
  causes, 88
  hyperphosphatemia and, 110, 113
  hypocalcemia and, 98
  hypocalcemia treatment and, 100
  indications, 20
  hypophosphatemia and, 21, 109, 112
  potassium and, 35, 80, 81, 85
Ringer's lactate, 34
RTA. *See* Renal tubular acidosis
RTC. *See* Cells, renal tubular

Salicylate poisoning
  dialysis and, 18
  metabolic acidosis and, 25, 26, 36, 86
  respiratory alkalosis and, 3, 51
Sarcoidosis, hypercalcemia in, 93
Sediment. *See* Cells, in urinary sediment
Serum chemistry, renal dysfunction and, 15 (table)
Serum glutamic oxaloacetic transaminase (SGOT), 21
  in differential diagnosis, 88
SIADH. *See* Syndrome of inappropriate antidiuretic hormone secretion
Sickle cell disease
  nephrogenic DI and, 71
  OU and, 11 (table)
  potassium deficiency and, 80, 81
Sodium
  serum
    in differential diagnosis, 15 (table), 50
    in hyperosmolar states, 73
    in hyponatremia, 59–60 (table), 62, 64, 65, 66, 84, 85
    in ketonemia assessment, 4
    in metabolic acidosis, 36, 40
    in metabolic alkalosis, 45, 46, 54
    in pseudohyponatremia, 57, 58
    in SIADH, 64
  total body
    in hyperosmolar states, 69, 70 (table)
    in hyponatremia, 59, 61

Sodium, total body—*Continued*
   in metabolic acidosis, 34, 39
   restriction, in ARF, 17, 18
  urine
   in ARF, 21, 22
   in differential diagnosis, 15 (table), 50
   in hyperosmolar states, 73
   in hyponatremia, 60, 66, 88
   in metabolic alkalosis, 44
   in RTA, 32
Sodium chloride
  in metabolic alkalosis, 46
  -responsive metabolic alkalosis, 44–45
  -unresponsive metabolic alkalosis, 44, 45
Specific gravity
  compared to osmolality, 2
  proteinuria, 3
Syndrome of inappropriate antidiuretic hormone secretion (SIADH)
  abnormal CSF and, 66
  causes, 60–61
  CNS disorder and, 85
  diagnostic criteria, 60
  hyponatremia and, 64
  modes of therapy, 61–62
Systemic lupus erythematosus, potassium deficiency and, 80, 81

Tamm-Horsfall protein, 3, 6
Tetany
  hypocalcemia and, 99–100
  hypomagnesemia and, 116
Thiazide diuretics. *See* Diuretics
Thyroid gland
  hypercalcemia and hyperthyroidism, 94, 103
  hyponatremia in hypothyroidism, 59
TRH. *See* Hormone, thyrotropin-releasing
Triglycerides, pseudohyponatremia and, 58
TRP. *See* Tubular reabsorption of phosphorus
TSH. *See* Hormone, thyroid-stimulating
Tuberculosis, hyponatremia and, 64
Tuberous sclerosis, 16
Tubules
  distal, 27, 28
  potassium loss in RTA, 78, 88
  proximal, 26 (table), 27, 28
Tubular reabsorption of phosphorus (TRP), 95

Tumor
  cell breakdown, potassium and, 81
  osteoblastic
   hypercalcemia and, 98
   hypocalcemia and, 98

Urea clearance, 13
Uremia. *See* Renal failure
Uric acid
  in diagnosis, 7
  dialysis, in ARF, 22
  in hyperphosphatemia, 113
  in proximal RTA, 29
Urinalysis, renal dysfunction and, 14 (table)
Urinary tract obstruction. *See* Obstructive uropathy (OU)
Urine
  acidification, 2
  color, pathologic causes, 2
  concentration
   chloride, in metabolic alkalosis, 44, 50
   in hypokalemia, 79
   in SIADH, 60
   sodium, in hyponatremia, 60, 66
   urinalysis and, 2
  dipstick test, 2, 3, 5
  osmolality. *See* Osmolality
  volume
   in ARF, 11 (table), 22
   furosemide therapy and, 21, 66
   in hypercalcemia, 97
   in hyperosmolar states, 71, 73
   in hyperphosphatemia, 114
   in hyponatremia, 60, 65
   mannitol therapy and, 21
Urine chemistry
  ARF and, 16
  PRA and, 16
Urine pH
  in acidemia, 28
  dipstick test, 2
  information obtainable from, 2
  proximal RTA and, 33
  RTA and, 32
  in urinary tract disease, 3

Vasopressin
  effect on DI, 71
  hyponatremia and, 59, 65
Vitamin A intoxication, and hypercalcemia, 94, 95
Vitamin D
  calcium homeostasis and, 92–93
  deficiency
   hypocalcemia and, 98, 99
   osteomalacia and, 99

functions, 93
human production of, 93
in intestinal absorption of calcium and phosphorus, 92, 93
intoxication, and hypercalcemia, 94, 103
metabolism of, abnormal, 98
overdose, hypercalcemia and, 94
therapy and, 97

Vomiting
hypokalemia and, 46
hyponatremia and, 59 (table)
metabolic alkalosis and, 44, 45, 47, 50, 55
potassium loss and, 77, 78

Water
dehydration, in hypernatremia, 70
in hyponatremia
brain content of, 74, 75
total body, 66
quantitation of excretion, 64, 73
restriction of, in ARF, 17